Chikungunya Virus - A Growing Global Public Health Threat

Edited by Jean Engohang-Ndong

Published in London, United Kingdom

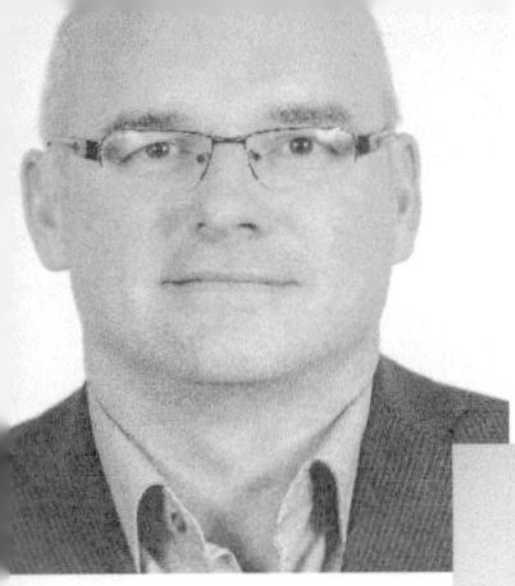
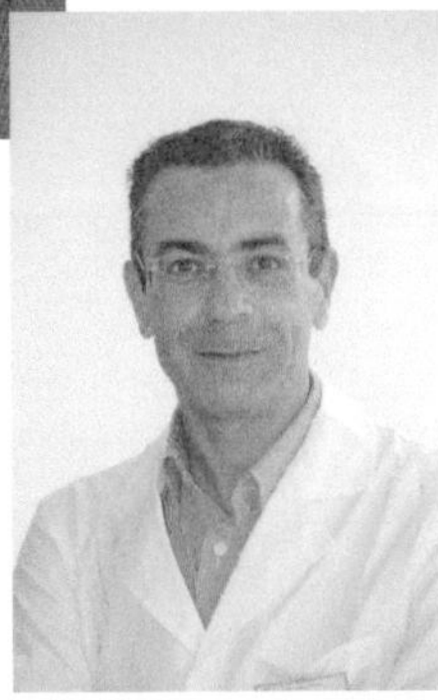
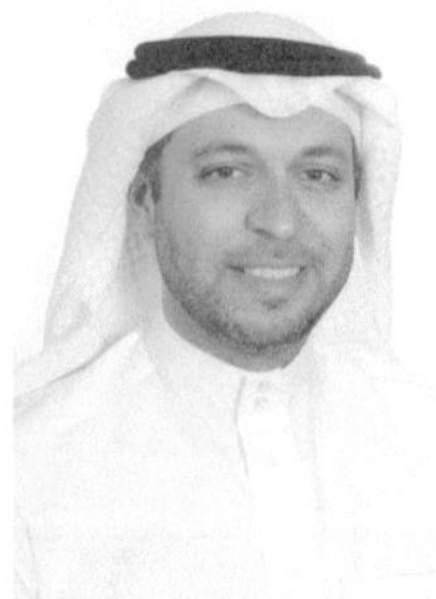
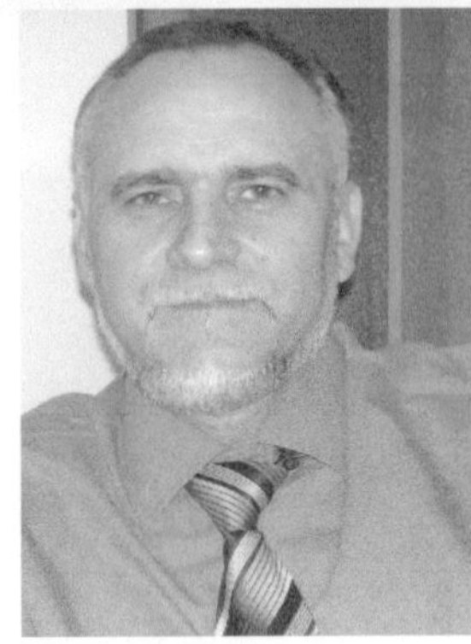
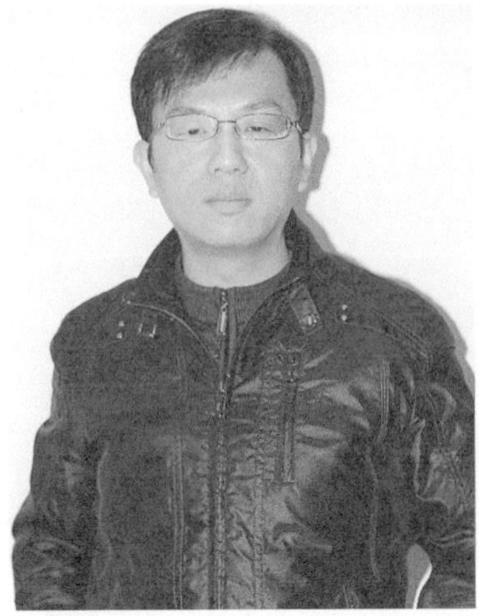
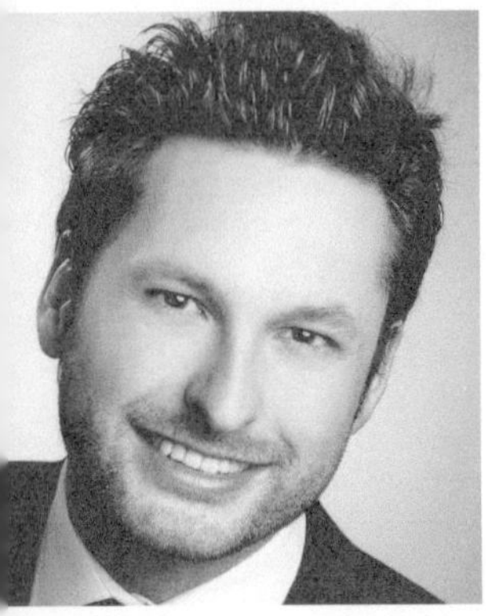
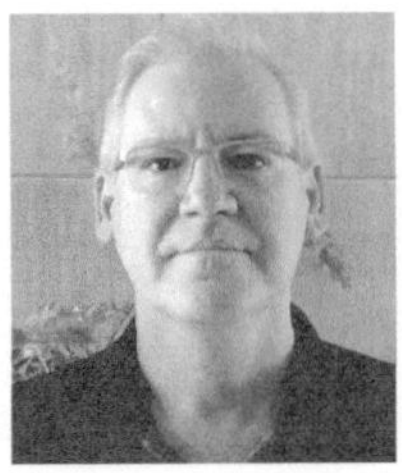

IntechOpen

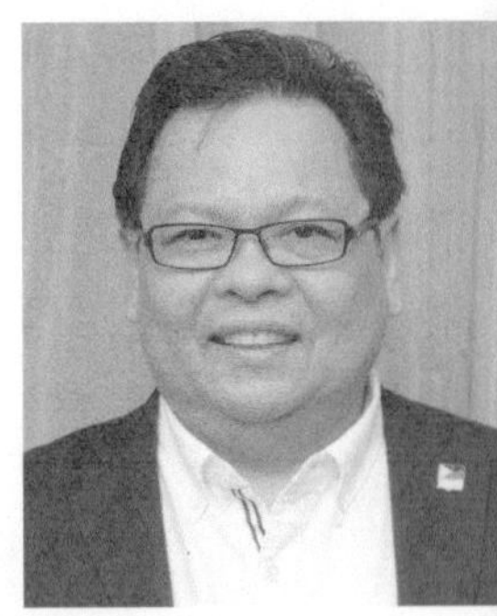
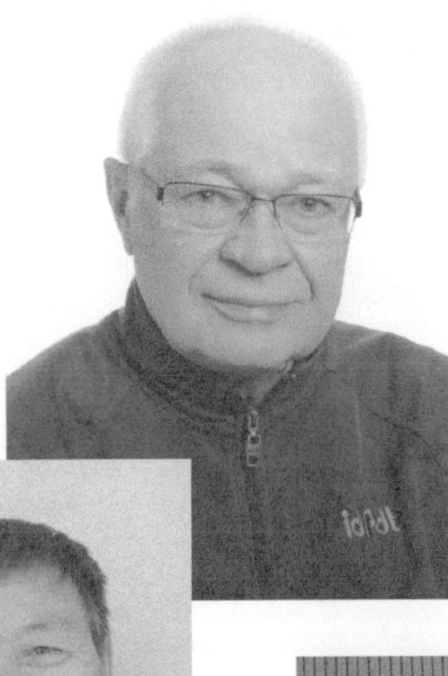
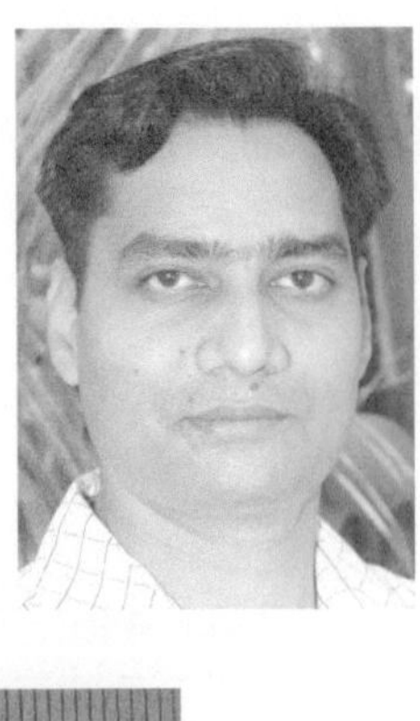
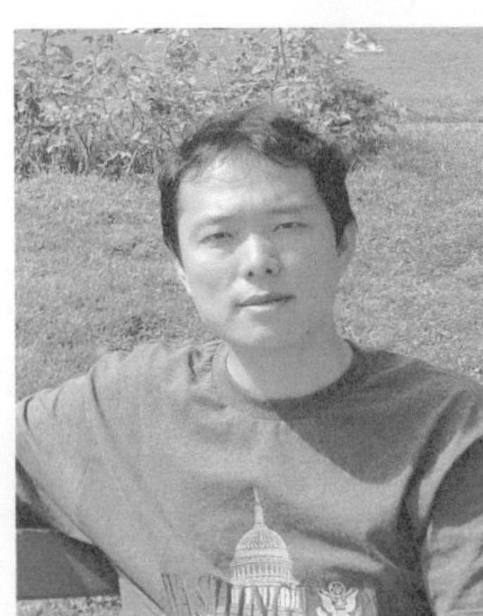
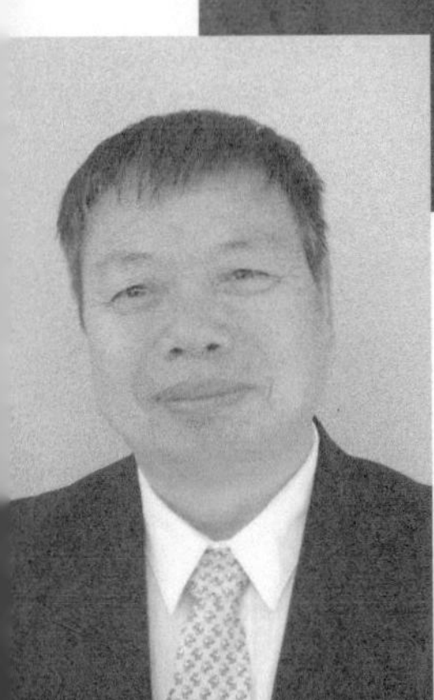
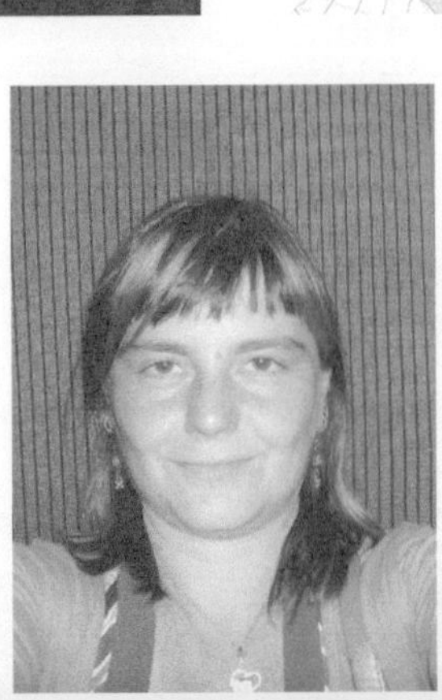

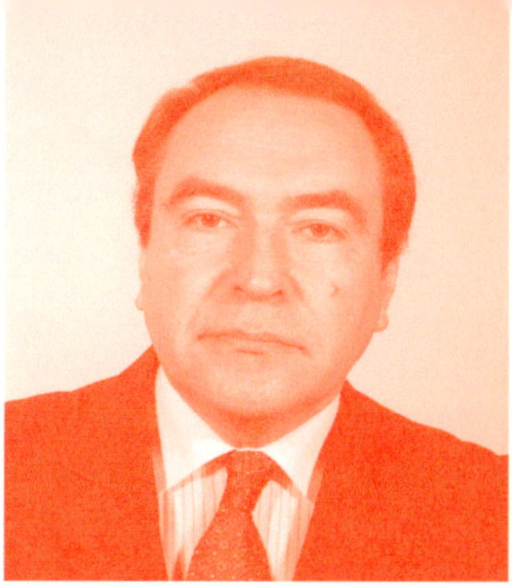
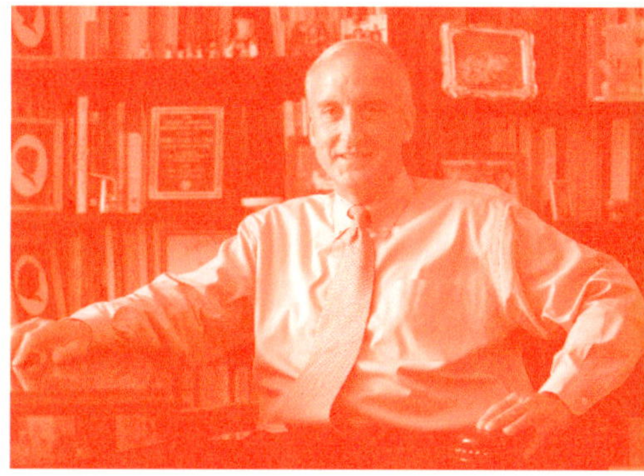
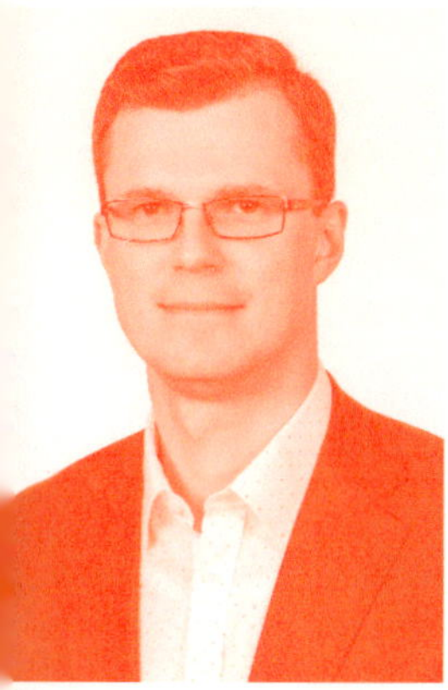
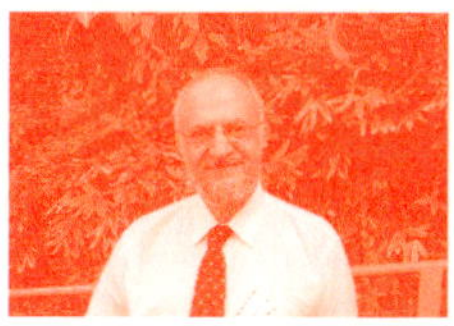
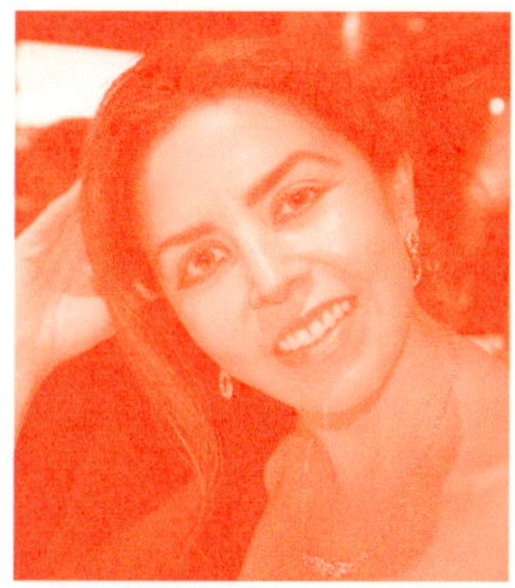

Supporting open minds since 2005

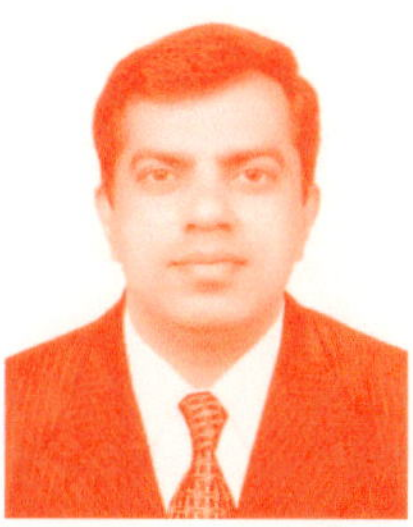
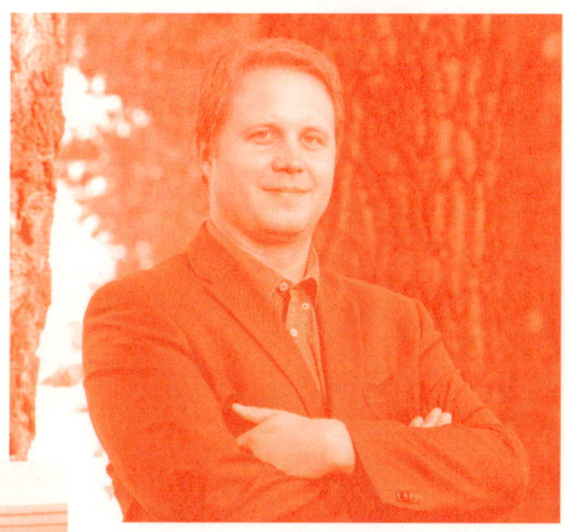
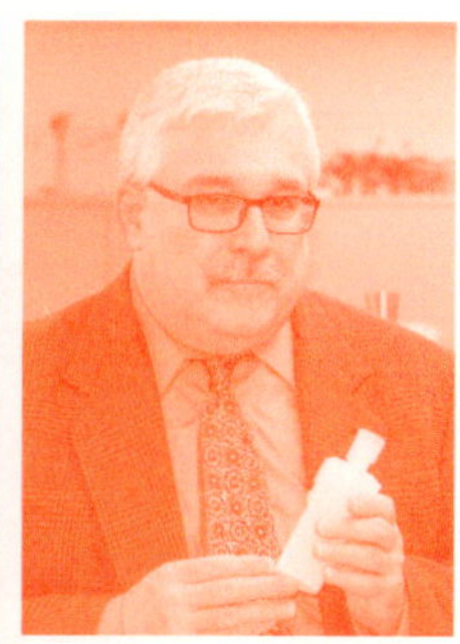
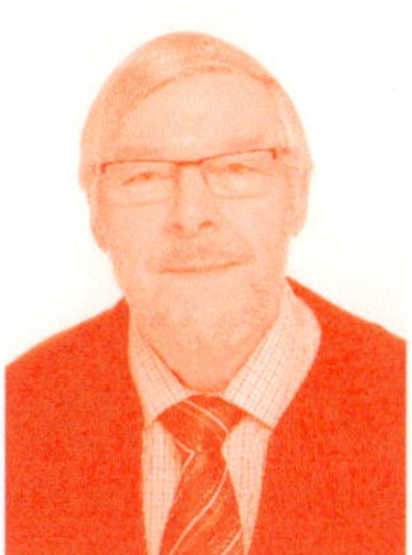
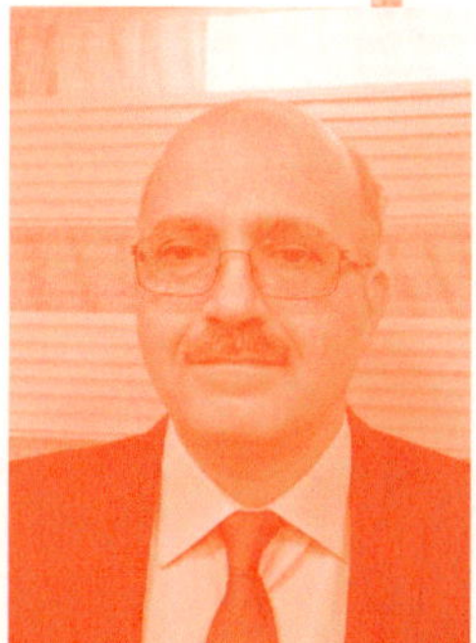
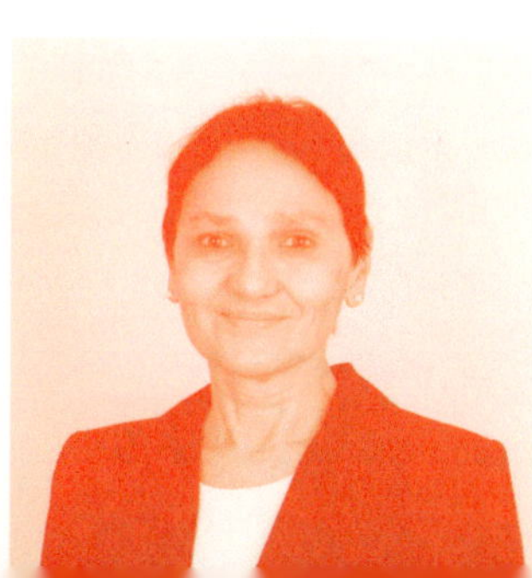
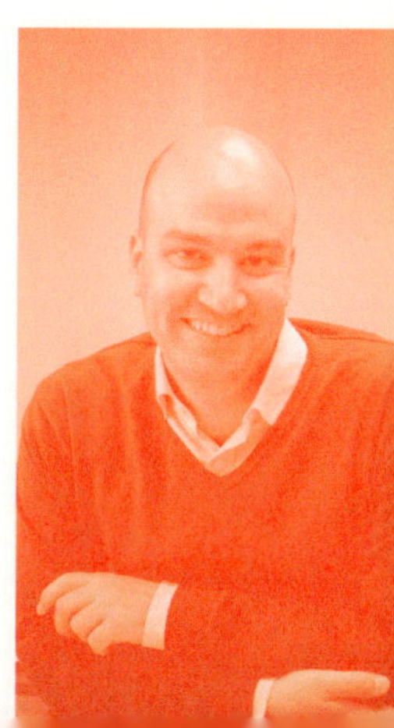

Chikungunya Virus - A Growing Global Public Health Threat
http://dx.doi.org/10.5772/intechopen.87411
Edited by Jean Engohang-Ndong

Part of IntechOpen Book Series: Infectious Diseases, Volume 12
Book Series Editor: Shailendra K. Saxena

Contributors
Fleury Augustin Nsole Biteghe, Tahir. B Dar, Chalomie Nyangone Ekome Toung, Arnaud John Kombe, Jean De La Croix Ndong, Neelakshi Mungra, Lucile Lyaruu, Juan A. Gonzalez-Sanchez, Maria Zavala-Colon, Tri Baskoro Tunggul Satoto, Nur Alvira Pascawati, Merhawi Debesai Oqbazgi, Jean Engohang-Ndong

First published in London, United Kingdom, 2022 by IntechOpen
IntechOpen is the global imprint of INTECHOPEN LIMITED, registered in England and Wales, registration number: 11086078, 5 Princes Gate Court, London, SW7 2QJ, United Kingdom
Printed in Croatia

British Library Cataloguing-in-Publication Data
A catalogue record for this book is available from the British Library

Additional hard and PDF copies can be obtained from orders@intechopen.com

Chikungunya Virus - A Growing Global Public Health Threat
Edited by Jean Engohang-Ndong
p. cm.
Print ISBN 978-1-83969-089-1
Online ISBN 978-1-83969-090-7
eBook (PDF) ISBN 978-1-83969-091-4
ISSN 2631-6188

For EU product safety concerns:
IN TECH d.o.o., Prolaz Marije Krucifikse Kozulić 3, 51000 Rijeka, Croatia, info@intechopen.com or visit our website at intechopen.com.

IntechOpen Book Series

Infectious Diseases

Volume 12

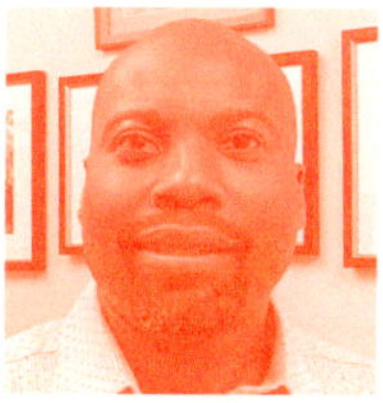

Dr. Jean Engohang-Ndong was born and raised in Gabon. After obtaining his Associate Degree of Science at the University of Science and Technology of Masuku, Gabon, he continued his education in France where he obtained his BS, MS, and Ph.D. in Medical Microbiology. He worked as a post-doctoral fellow at the Public Health Research Institute (PHRI), Newark, NJ for four years before accepting a three-year faculty position at Brigham Young University-Hawaii. Dr. Engohang-Ndong is a tenured faculty member with the academic rank of Full Professor at Kent State University, Ohio, where he teaches a wide range of biological science courses and pursues his research in medical and environmental microbiology. Recently, he expanded his research interest to epidemiology and biostatistics of chronic diseases in Gabon.

Editor of Volume 12:
Jean Engohang-Ndong
Department of Biological Sciences, Kent State University at Tuscarawas
New Philadelphia, Ohio, United States of America

Book Series Editor:
Shailendra K. Saxena
King George's Medical University

Scope of the Series

The series will give a most comprehensive overview of recent trends in various infectious diseases (as per the most recent Baltimore classification), as well as general concepts of infections, immunopathology, diagnosis, treatment, epidemiology and etiology to current clinical recommendations in management of infectious diseases, highlighting the ongoing issues, recent advances, with future directions in diagnostic approaches and therapeutic strategies. This book series will focus on various aspects and properties of infectious diseases whose deep understanding is very important for safeguarding human race from more loss of resources and economies due to pathogens.

Contents

Preface

Our current understanding of the microbial world and its role in human health has allowed microbiologists to determine the involvement of viruses in human health. Many diseases afflicting humankind are caused by viruses. As I write these words, for exactly two years month for month, the face of the entire world has turned completely inside out, affecting all aspects of our lives and our institutions due to a viral infection: the coronavirus disease caused by SARS-CoV-2 or COVID-19. From our social interactions to our professional routines that have completely changed, global trades and the world economy have all been so much disturbed that it is nearly impossible for any expert to say with certainty when our social interactions, professional lives, international trades, and the world economy will go back to "normal." Due to the coronavirus pandemic, the only certainty we have at this point is the uncertainty of tomorrow. While COVID-19 is an extreme case of viral infection, some more mild are silently disturbing the lives of many hundreds of thousands of people and families across the globe. It is the case of the chikungunya virus that causes chikungunya fever, which is endemic to tropical forested and subtropical areas of the globe. More recently, the virus has spilled over into temperate regions of the globe. Interestingly, despite the continual spread of the disease to new regions of the world where the disease was not observed or described before, chikungunya fever remains nevertheless unknown to not only the lay public but also and shockingly to even seasoned health professionals. The extreme difficulty for most people including health professionals, patients, and their families to tell chikungunya fever apart from some other viral infections such as dengue fever and Zika fever because of the extreme similarity of clinical symptoms exhibited between these three diseases prompted me to take on the challenge to serve as the academic editor of this book.

Hence, as I was invited to serve as the academic editor and started the work on this book, I had in mind four major audiences: health professionals, scientific investigators, patients, and the curious reader.

Health professionals, physicians and nurses alike, are at the forefront of the fight against chikungunya fever. Therefore, it is important to me to provide them with essential information necessary for a correct diagnosis of the disease at an early stage of onset. Misdiagnosis caused by the lack of education of health professionals even in endemic countries often leads to the unnecessary suffering of patients. Sometimes, unfortunately, the disease evolves into complicated forms. Thus, a major goal of mine was to keep health professionals informed about innovative tools and modern approaches currently available and/or in an advanced stage of investigation for them to unambiguously achieve a diagnosis of chikungunya fever in a timely manner when patients turn to them for care.

For young scientific investigators interested in studying the chikungunya virus, a book that covers broad aspects of the disease such as its history, epidemiology, spread and pathogenesis, and new perspectives in the pipeline for its prevention and treatment, represents a one-stop-shop for initiating and/or enriching a research topic on the disease. While there is currently no antiviral drug available to treat the disease, young investigators will learn about new promising drugs currently in the pipeline. These promising drugs, some of which are already in clinical trials, may constitute a starting point for more advanced research on drug discovery to treat the chikungunya virus. Moreover, young researchers will learn about the work being done on the development of a vaccine and other sophisticated approaches actively under investigation to prevent the spread of the infection across the globe.

While working on this book, my thoughts went also to patients and families of patients. Patients and their families are the first victims of the disease. So, as chikungunya fever spreads around the world, educating patients, their families, and populations at risk of the disease and its impact on the quality of life of patients seemed important to me. Helping patients understand the nature of the infection and how their life may be affected in the short and/or long term is important for them and their families to know what to expect and with that knowledge, be prepared to seek adequate support to alleviate suffering.

For populations at risk of exposure to the chikungunya virus, the information contained in this book is valuable in that it will help them take appropriate measures to reduce the chances of infection.

The speed of globalization of exchanges, in the context of the 21st century, forces us to be curious about what is happening across the world, regardless of where we live and where we travel to. The impact of the COVID-19 pandemic on our lives has taught us to be considerate of what is going on around the globe. Thus, it is more and more crucial to be curious and have a good idea about potential public health threats such as chikungunya fever. While going through this book, the curious reader will learn about the chikungunya virus, the public health threat it represents, and what is being done to counteract its spread and limit its chance of becoming a pandemic.

Jean Engohang-Ndong
Department of Biological Sciences,
Kent State University at Tuscarawas,
New Philadelphia, Ohio, United States of America

Section 1

Introduction to Chikungunya

Chapter 1

Introductory Chapter: Introduction to Chikungunya

Jean Engohang-Ndong

1. Introduction to chikungunya

The "Golden Age of Microbiology" that spanned from roughly 1857 through 1914 was not only marked by the identification of many bacterial infectious agents that ravaged the lives of millions of people across the world with *Mycobacterium tuberculosis*, the causative agent of human tuberculosis being one of the most dreaded infectious bacteria discovered at the time, that period was also very special because the work on viruses started. Indeed, in 1892, Dmitri Ivanosky discovered that the sap of diseased tobacco plants could infect healthy tobacco plants even after passing the sap through a Chamberland's porcelain filter which was typically used to trap bacteria. While Dmitri hypothesized that his results could be the consequence of cracked filters, Martinus Beijerinck demonstrated in 1898 that what he called *Contagium vivum fluidum* (contagious living fluid in Latin) contained infectious particles which size was much smaller than bacteria in such a way that they could persist in the filtrate through the Chamberland's porcelain filters. Later, the discovery and partial characterization of bacteriophages opened new avenues for the explosion of the study of viruses.

The invention of the electron microscope in 1931 revolutionized the study of viruses when for the first time, bacteriophages were shown to have a very complex structural organization. As microscopy evolved to unravel the tremendous diversity of the viral world, the progress in molecular biology, biochemistry, and biophysics allowed the development of a structural model that led to the characterization of not only bacteriophages and plant viruses, but also animal viruses including the influenza virus, the poliovirus, and the Epstein-Barr virus to name only those.

The second half of the 20th century marked the discovery of over 2000 bacterial, plant, and animal viruses. Among the human virus newly discovered was the chikungunya virus (CHIKV) which is the etiologic agent of the chikungunya fever (CHIKF) and was discovered in Tanzania in the 1950s [1]. CHIKV which belongs to the *Togaviridae* family and to the genus of *Alphavirus*, is known to cause fever and joint pain that wear off within a week in most patients. However, in some patients, the joint pain may linger for months and/or eventually lead to arthralgia. Other symptoms may include headaches, myalgia also known as muscle pain, joint swelling, or rash. The next few paragraphs of this chapter and subsequent chapters of this book will explore the organization of the virus, the history of the disease it causes, its epidemiology, the current treatment status, and perspectives for new treatment and prevention of the disease.

2. Genomic and structural organization of the chikungunya virus

Since its discovery in the 1950s, CHIKV has been relatively well characterized, with a clear description of its genomic makeup and its structural organization (**Figure 1**).

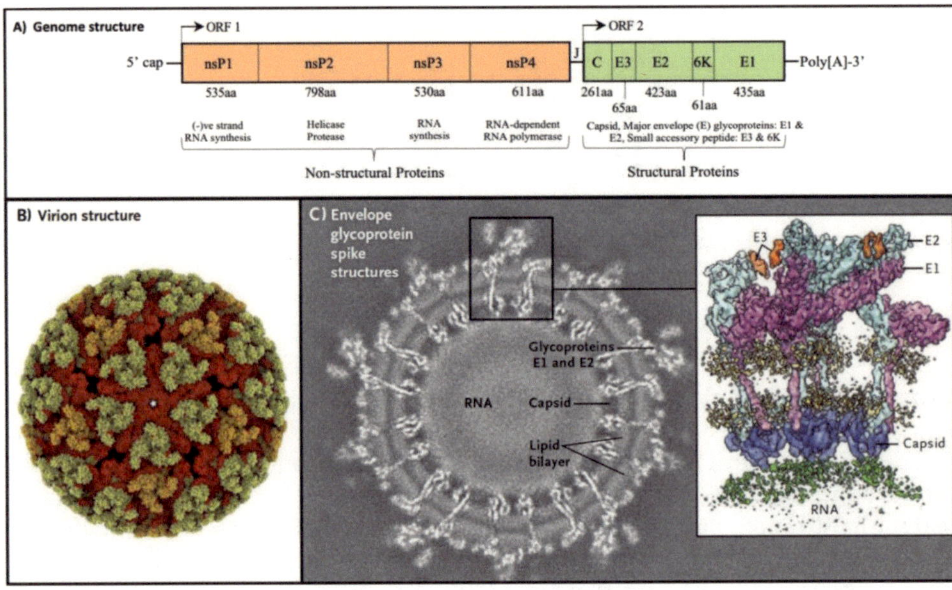

Figure 1.
Chikungunya virus genomic and structural organizations. (A) The genomic organization of CHIKV shows two groups of genes, including genes encoding non-structural proteins (NsP1-4) and genes encoding structural proteins C (capsid), E1 and E2 (envelope glycoproteins), and E3 and 6 K which are small accessory polypeptides. (B) 3D reconstruction of CHIKV showing the E1 basal triangle (red) and the E2 protrusion for each spike (green and yellow). (C) Shows spike-protein predicted structures based on atomic resolution structures of the envelope glycoproteins and high-resolution cryo-electron microscopic reconstructions of CHIKV [2, 3].

Thus, like many other alphaviruses, full genome sequencing and cryo-electron microscopic reconstruction [2] revealed that CHIV is a small, spherical, enveloped virus with a genome of about 11.8 kb composed of a single-strand positive RNA flanked at its 5′- and 3′-extremities with untranslated regions (UTR). The role of these UTRs is to regulate important biological functions such as viral replication, transcription, and viral packaging during a lytic cycle. The 5′-UTR is preceded by a cap while the 3′-UTR is followed by a poly[A] tail. The cap and the poly[A] tail are both responsible for protecting the core information of the viral genome from the damaging effects of exonucleases. *In vitro* molecular and *in silico* analyses of the structural organization of the genome reveal that the CHIKV genome contains two open reading frames, ORF 1 and ORF 2 which are connected through a small polynucleotide sequence that is untranslated. That polynucleotide sequence constitutes a junction sequence (**Figure 1A**).

ORF 1 which is located at the 5′ end of the genome carries four genes which expression leads to the production of four non-structural proteins called NsP1, NsP2, NsP3, and NsP4. More specifically, CHIKV NsP1 is a viral capping enzyme while CHIKV NsP2 contains ATPase, RNA triphosphatase, helicase, and protease activities [4]. The two other CHIKV NsPs exhibit ADP-ribose-1-phosphate phosphatase and RNA-binding activities for NsP3 and RNA-dependent RNA-polymerase activity for CHIKV NsP4 [5]. These four non-structural proteins are essential for the replication of the viral genome during the infection cycle.

ORF 2 which is situated at the 3′ end of the genome arbores the five genes encoding five structural proteins including C, the capsid protein that forms a protective coat around the positive-RNA genome; E1 and E2, the two envelope glycoproteins, which both form the spikes on the surface of virion particles, and E3 and 6 K which are two small accessory proteins of the envelope. The viral spike proteins facilitate attachment to cell surfaces and entry of viral particles into the host cell.

Using advanced imaging technology such as atomic resolution and cryo-electron microscopy, research teams have been able to reconstruct the three-dimensional organization of CHIKV and the fine structures of the viral envelope (**Figure 1B** and **C**). That imaging resolution of CHIKV shows that both E1 and E2 form a heterodimer in which both glycoproteins are intertwined and form the spikes on the surface of the virus. E1 and E2 have transmembrane domains that span the phospholipid bilayer of the viral membrane. The endodomains of both proteins interact with the capsid protein while the ectodomains of E1 and E2 that are also glycosylated make up the spikes which are suspected to be the receptor-binding domains responsible for attachment and entry of the virion into host cells [2, 3, 6].

3. Global threat

It is now well established that since its discovery in Tanzania, CHIKV has been in circulation across the world and virtually in all continents including in Africa, in Asia, the Indian subcontinent, the Americas, and in Europe (**Figure 2**). It is thought that the virus circulated initially and primarily in sylvatic regions of sub-Saharan Africa in a cycle involving non-human primates and arboreal mosquito species of the *Aedes* genus as vectors. During the heavy rainy season, sylvatic mosquitoes multiply to the point that they would spread into villages and/or urban centers surrounding the rainforests where the arthropod could now infect human subjects. Following the enzootic sylvatic cycle and the human village cycle, the migration of villagers to urban centers and cities could lead to the spread of the infectious agents to humans living in these cities where the transmission cycle would now involve the urban mosquitos *Aedes aegypti* and/or *A. albopictus*. Spillover of mosquito vectors from villages to urbanized centers can also lead to the translocation of the infection to urban centers. Spillover infections have been documented in many African countries including, but not limited to Cameroon, Senegal, South Africa, and Zimbabwe. From Africa, the chikungunya virus has now spread to Asia, Australia, Europe, India, and the Americas. In the Americas,

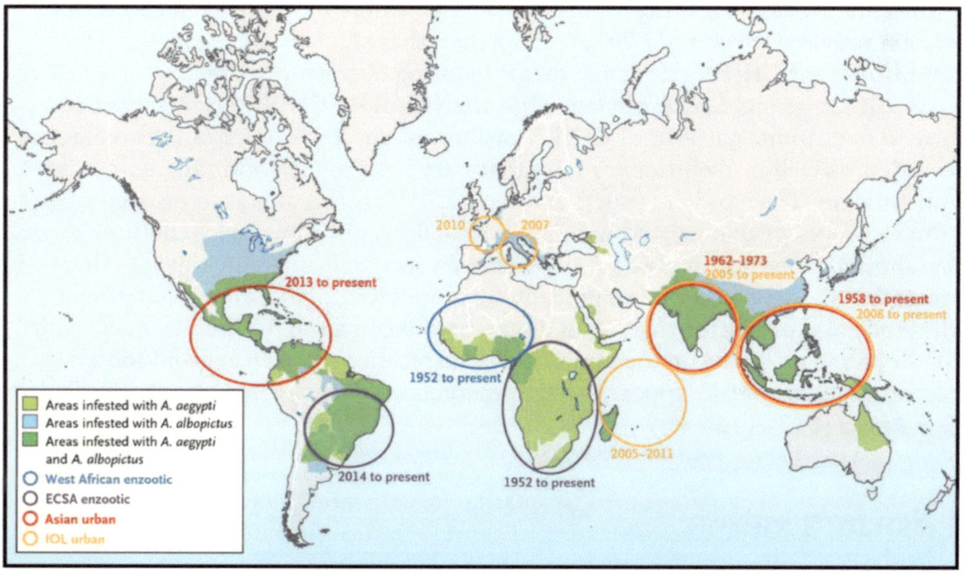

Figure 2.
The spread of the chikungunya virus across the globe between the time of its discovery to the present [7].

the disease has been found in southern states of the United States of America and in many countries of South America. Two major strains of the virus have been circulating in Africa: the eastern, central, southern African enzootic (ECSA) strain and the West African enzootic strain. Out of all the chikungunya virus strains found in circulation in the world, only ECSA and the west African strains involve a sylvatic cycle. Between 1958 and 1973, new CHIKV strains emerged as Asian strains in an urban cycle in many Asian countries, in India and a myriad of islands distributed between the south china sea and the Indian Ocean. In 2005, new outbreaks of the chikungunya fever emerged in the Indian ocean and in Asia. The CHIKV strain responsible for that outbreak was only involved in an urban cycle and never in a sylvatic cycle. Eventually, that Indian ocean strain spread to some parts of Africa and Europe including in France and Italy. More recently, the ECSA enzootic strain of CHIKV spread to South America while the Asian urban CHIKV strain spread to the two hemispheres of the American continent. Due to the ubiquity of air transport throughout the world, air travelers arriving from endemic areas to new territories contributed to the establishment and the spread of the chikungunya fever. Ultimately, new strains carried around the world including in Europe and in the Americas started circulating in local transmission.

The unusually dramatic increase in the incidence of the disease worldwide during the past decade could be explained by multiple factors including, but not limited to the improvement of transport means and increase of air travel which opened ways for a quick spread of the disease between continents; the expansion of urban areas in tropical regions of Africa and South America that were previously forested; the increased density in urban areas of human population and mosquito population of the genus *Aedes*; the new exposure of the of south Asian and the Indian basin populations to the vector of the virus. In addition to *A. aegypti*, since the mid-1980s, the invasion of the species *A. albopictus* which is known to be the major second CHIKV vector from Asia where it originated into surrounding continental countries and islands in the Indian Ocean basin, Africa, and southern Europe was made possible by a constantly growing global trade. Furthermore, the current increase in global temperature and subsequent projections of climate change will only exacerbate the spread of both *A. aegypti* and *A. albopictus*, therefore, a spread of the chikungunya virus to regions of the globe where the arthropod genus *Aedes* was not previously endemic. Taken altogether, these factors are creating perfect conditions for a CHIKV pandemic that is looming over the horizon.

In 2010, a genome-scale phylogenetic analysis of 40 CHIKV strains was performed to examine patterns of CHIKV evolution, and the origins of outbreaks recorded, as well as evolutionary rates that vary between enzootic and epidemic transmission. That study revealed that the CHIKV strains analyzed evolved from a common ancestor that existed within the last 500 years. The phylogenetic analysis also showed some geographic overlap between two main enzootic lineages that were previously thought to be geographically separated within the African continent. The study also estimated that CHIKV was introduced from Africa into Asia about 70–90 years ago. Based on the same study, the recent Indian Ocean and Indian subcontinent outbreaks appear to have emerged independently from continental East Africa [6].

4. New perspectives

The fight against the chikungunya virus has been arduous. However, despite that hard work and many accomplishments, a lot of work still remains to be done in many areas, including in prevention, diagnosis, and treatment of the disease.

4.1 Prevention

The golden approach to control an infection is to limit as much as possible exposure of sensitive subjects to the infectious agent. In the case of the chikungunya fever, a control of the proliferation of mosquito vectors and the development of a vaccine are two approaches the are being actively considered. In 2013, a team of researchers in Italy developed a cost-effective sterile insect technique with the final goal to suppress *A. albopictus* populations. *A. albopictus* is known to widely proliferate in man-made containers such as tires, buckets, and barrels with a high proportion of urban and suburban distribution. These two features made possible the application of the sterile insect control strategies. Thus, males *A. albopictus* were irradiated with gamma rays and released in the field. The adult population density was estimated by monitoring egg production in the ovitraps, while the radiation induced sterility was estimated by measuring the hatching percentage of weekly collected eggs in sterile insect technique and control sites. These experiments revealed that sterile males released at the rate of 896–1590 males per hectare per week led to a remarkable sterility level in the local population. Likewise, a high level of sterility led to an important decrease of the egg density in the ovitraps. Taken together, these two findings allowed researchers to formulate the assumption that if egg sterility values of at least 80% are achieved, that level should be enough to secure a suppression of the local population of mosquitoes [8]. While trials of control of mosquito populations using sterile insect technique is promising, it is nevertheless important to consider the immigration of mated females in the areas where sterilization of male mosquitoes was pursued. Therefore, combining sterilization of male mosquitoes along with an application of traditional population control methods such as the management of standing water or the application of insecticides is highly recommended.

In addition to innovative mosquito vector population control methods, a French company called Valneva SE recently developed a promising chikungunya vaccine to prevent the disease. In 2020, Valneva announced the initiation of a pivotal phase 3 clinical trial for its single-shot chikungunya vaccine candidate VLA1553. The promising chikungunya vaccine candidate VLA1553 is a live-attenuated CHIKV which was made mild by deleting a large part of the gene encoding the non-structural protein NsP3 [9]. This vaccine candidate was designed to prevent outbreaks and to provide protection against various CHIKV phylogroups and various CHIKV strains. The phase 3 clinical trial was conducted in the United States of America across 44 sites and involved 4115 adults which ages were 18 years and older. After a single shot, analysis of the serum of participants 28 days after inoculation of the candidate vaccine revealed that the vaccine induced a 98.5% protection in participants. Furthermore, when assessed for safety, results indicated that the CHIKV vaccine candidate VLA1553 was well tolerated by 3082 participants [10].

4.2 Diagnosis

Chikungunya fever, dengue fever, and the Zika fever are all caused by mosquitoes from the *Aedes* genus. The three diseases are characterized by an onset of fever, arthralgia, myalgia, and rash. That extreme similarity of symptoms between these different diseases leads most of the time and unfortunately to misdiagnosis and prescription of inappropriate treatment to patients. The lack of early accurate diagnosis of the disease may cause an evolution of the disease to complicated forms much more deleterious to the patient. The recent development of molecular diagnosis tools has opened new avenues for accurate diagnosis of the chikungunya fever and to tell it apart from the dengue virus infection or the Zika fever. The primary laboratory test used to detect CHIKV or viral RNA is the analysis of the patient serum collected less than 6 days after the onset of the disease through a molecular biology approach called real-time reverse transcription polymerase chain reaction (RT-PCR). Real time RT-PCR is a laboratory technique of molecular biology commonly used for detecting the presence of specific genetic material of infectious agents including viruses. Originally, the RT-PCR technique used radioactive isotopes such as ^{32}P to detect targeted genetic materials, but in the past two decades, the technique has been refined and radioisotopes have been progressively replaced by fluorescent dyes which are safer for the user and much more environmentally friendly. Real time RT-PCR allows researchers to see the results almost immediately while the reaction is still in progress. That approach was used by Bandeira and colleagues when they reported the presence of CHIKV RNA in the blood, urine, and semen during the acute phase of the disease in an adult patient with dengue virus (DENV) type 3 co-infection [11]. In that particular case, patient samples were first submitted to viral RNA extraction procedure followed by real time RT-PCR to screen for CHIKV, DENV, and the zika virus. Besides the real time RT-PCR technique, the second most reliable approach is by seeking CHIKV-specific immunoglobulin M (IgM) in patient samples. IgM detection is possible for sample collected roughly more than 5 days after the onset of the ailment [12, 13]. Thus, serological diagnosis makes it possible for physicians both experienced and young practitioners to draw a clear distinction between the chikungunya fever, the dengue fever, and the Zika virus infection and to develop an unambiguous diagnosis of the disease. It is worth noting however that the limited access to these two state-of-the art diagnosis approaches in remote rural, semi-urban, and urban endemic regions in countries where resources are not equally distributed still represents a huge obstacle to a systematic clear diagnosis of the chikungunya fever.

4.3 Treatment

To this day, there is no medicine approved by government agencies or international organizations such as the World Health Organization to treat CHIKV infection. Treatments commonly used during the course of CHIKV infection are typically geared toward the relief of symptoms such as fever and pain. Nonsteroidal anti-inflammatory drugs among which paracetamol, acetaminophen, and nibuprofen are often used to relieve symptoms of the disease. While not one single antiviral drug specifically directed against CHIKV has been approved, there are however several chemical components that have been investigated and stand as potential chemotherapeutic agents promising for the treatment of the chikungunya fever. Chloroquine for instance has shown to be effective against CHIKV through its obstructive activity against the entry of CHIKV into host cells [14]. Nevertheless, despite the promising *in vitro* results of that drug, clinical trials have failed to confirm any real benefit to patients. Similarly, suramin which has been approved by the Food and Drug Administration in the United State to treat trypanosomiasis which is caused by the protist *Trypanosoma brucei*, has also shown to be effective at preventing the entry of CHIKV in host cells during *in vitro* tests. Interestingly, while suramin is an effective anti-CHIKV drug *in vitro*, the adverse effects induced by the drug out weight the benefit to patients as the chikungunya fever remains mild in most patients. Multiple modified versions of suramin or suramin conjugates have shown promising results *in vivo* against CHIKV infection [15].

In addition to inhibitors of CHIV entry into the host cell, other promising anti-CHIKV have been identified and grouped based on their mode of action. Thus, some anti-CHIKV have shown to be NsP1 inhibitors, NsP2 inhibitors, and

Compounds	Mechanism of action
Chloroquine	CHIKV entry inhibitors
Suramin conjugates	
Lobaric acid	nsP1 inhibitors
Bassettos *in silico* lead (compound 1)	nsP2 inhibitors
Ribavirin	nsP4 inhibitors and inhibitors of viral genome replication
b-d-N4-hydroxycytidine (NHC)	
Prostratin	Protein kinase C inhibitors
12-O-tetradecanoylphorbol 13-acetate (TPA)	
Phorbol-12,13-didecanoate	
12-O-decanoylphorbol 13-acetate (DPA)	
12-O-decanoyl-7-hydroperoxy-5-ene-13-acetate	
Phorbol	
Neoguillauminin A	
12-deoxy phorbol (compound 1)	
12-deoxyphorbol (compound 2)	
12-deoxyphorbol (compound 4)	
Trigocherrin A	

Table 1.
Selected promising anti-CHIKV compounds [14].

NsP4 inhibitors while others exhibit an ability to inhibit the replication of the virus genome. Finally, some plant extracts harvested from the *Euphobiaceae* family with protein kinase C inhibitory activity also show strong anti-CHIKV activity (**Table 1**).

5. Conclusion

The chikungunya fever which is caused by a virus of the *Togaviridae* family, is characterized by the development of fever, and join pain. While the disease is rarely fetal, it can however evolve into severe arthralgia and myalgia. The development of modern molecular tools and atomic microscope tools have allowed scientists to achieve the sequencing and annotation of the virus complete genome and the resolution of the chikungunya virus structure. Thus, it is established that CHIKV is an enveloped virus with spikes that allow that bioparticle to attach to receptors located on the surface of host cells. CHIKV is not only occurring in tropical regions of Africa and south America, but it has also spread to other regions beyond the tropics in such way that it has become a global public health issue that requires a global approach for controlling the spread of the disease. The extreme similarity of symptoms found between CHIKV infection and some other viral infections including the Zika virus infection and the dengue virus infection has made it necessary to develop diagnosis tools specific for the detection of CHIKV infection in patients. Research interests in the development of vaccines and the discovery of anti-CHIKV drugs have opened the way to a strong vaccine candidate and to anti-CHIKV drug candidates. Nevertheless, the battle for controlling the chikungunya fever is far from being over.

Conflict of interest

The authors declare no conflict of interest.

Author details

Jean Engohang-Ndong
Kent State University at Tuscarawas, New Philadelphia, OH, United States of America

*Address all correspondence to: jengohan@kent.edu

References

[1] Ross RW. The Newala epidemic. III. The virus: Isolation, pathogenic properties, and relationship to the epidemic. The Journal of Hygiene. 1956;**54**:177-191. DOI: 10.1017/S0022172400044442

[2] Zhang R, Hryc CF, Cong Y, Liu X, Jakana J, Gorchakov R, et al. 4.4 Å cryo-EM structure of an enveloped alphavirus Venezuelan equine encephalitis virus. The EMBO Journal. 2011;**30**(18):3854-3863. DOI: 10.1038/emboj.2011.261

[3] Voss JE, Vaney MC, Duquerroy S, Vonrhein C, Girard-Blanc C, Crublet E, et al. Glycoprotein organization of chikungunya virus particles revealed by X-ray crystallography. Nature. 2010; **468**(7324):709-712. DOI: 10.1038/nature09555

[4] Kumar S, Kumar A, Mamidi P, Tiwari A, Kumar S, Mayavannan A, et al. Chikungunya virus nsP1 interacts directly with nsP2 and modulates its ATPase activity. Scientific Reports. 2018;**8**(1):1045. DOI: 10.1038/s41598-018-19295-0

[5] Ahola T, Merits A. Functions of chikungunya virus nonstructural proteins. In: Chikungunya Virus: Advances in Biology, Pathogenesis, and Treatment. 2016. Cham: Springer International Publishing AG; pp. 75-98. DOI: 10.1007/978-3-319-42958-8_6

[6] Volk SM, Chen R, Tsetsarkin KA, Adams AP, Garcia TI, Sall AA, et al. Genome-scale phylogenetic analyses of chikungunya virus reveal independent emergences of recent epidemics and various evolutionary rates. Journal of Virology. 2010;**84**(13):6497-6504. DOI: 10.1128/JVI.01603-09

[7] Weaver SC, Lecuit M. Chikungunya virus and the global spread of a mosquito-borne disease. The New England Journal of Medicine. 2015;**372**(13):1231-1239. DOI: 10.1056/NEJMra1406035

[8] Bellini R, Medici A, Puggioli A, Balestrino F, Carrieri M. Pilot field trials with *Aedes albopictus* irradiated sterile males in Italian urban areas. Journal of Medical Entomology. 2013;**50**(2):317-325. DOI: 10.1603/me12048

[9] Hallengärd D, Kakoulidou M, Lulla A, Kümmerer BM, Johansson DX, Mutso M, et al. Novel attenuated chikungunya vaccine candidates elicit protective immunity in C57BL/6 mice. Journal of Virology. 2014;**88**(5):2858-2866. DOI: 10.1128/JVI.03453-13

[10] Valneva SE. Valneva announces positive phase 3 pivotal results for its single-shot chikungunya vaccine candidate. 2021. Available from: https://valneva.com/wp-content/uploads2021/08/2021_08_05_VLA1553_Phase3_Results_PR_EN.pdf [Accessed: 5 August 2021]

[11] Bandeira AC, Campos GS, Rocha VF, Souza BS, Soares MB, Oliveira AA, et al. Prolonged shedding of chikungunya virus in semen and urine: A new perspective for diagnosis and implications for transmission. IDCases. 2016;**6**:100-103. DOI: 10.1016/j.idcr.2016.10.007

[12] Cho B, Jeon BY, Kim J, Noh J, Kim J, Park M, et al. Expression and evaluation of chikungunya virus E1 and E2 envelope proteins for serodiagnosis of chikungunya virus infection. Yonsei Medical Journal. 2008;**49**(5):828-835. DOI: 10.3349/ymj.2008.49.5.828

[13] Johnson BW, Russell BJ, Goodman CH. Laboratory diagnosis of chikungunya virus infections and commercial sources for diagnostic assays. The Journal of Infectious Diseases. 2016;**214**(Suppl. 5):S471-S474. DOI: 10.1093/infdis/jiw274

[14] Hucke F, Bugert JJ. Current and promising antivirals against chikungunya virus. Frontiers in Public Health. 2020;**8**:618624. DOI: 10.3389/fpubh.2020.618624

[15] Hwu JR, Gupta NK, Tsay SC, Huang WC, Albulescu IC, Kovacikova K, et al. Bis(benzofuran-thiazolidinone)s and bis(benzofuran-thiazinanone)s as inhibiting agents for chikungunya virus. Antiviral Research. 2017;**146**:96-101. DOI: 10.1016/j.antiviral.2017.08.008

Section 2

History

Chapter 2

History and Geographic Distribution of Chikungunya Virus

Maria Zavala-Colon and Juan A. Gonzalez-Sanchez

Abstract

Chikungunya fever (CHIKF) is a mosquito-borne disease caused by an arbovirus endemic to Africa and Asia. It was initially seen in the early 1950s at the boundary of Tanzania and Mozambique. Due to the ease with which its vectors propagate, the virus has spread to India, Europe, and recently it arrived in the Caribbean, eventually extending into North, Central, and South America. According to the World Health Organization (WHO), the most common clinical manifestations are abrupt fever, polyarthralgia, headache, maculopapular rash, myalgia, and nausea/vomiting. Severe joint pain and stiffness have been known to incapacitate some patients from a few days to several months after infection. The re-emergence of the CHIKV and its spread to new places around the globe has encouraged the development of new preventive, diagnostic, and treatment strategies. This chapter will discuss the history of CHIKV and expanding geographic distribution.

Keywords: chikungunya virus, fever, *Aedes aegypti*, history, geography, outbreaks

1. Introduction

The chinkungunya virus (CHIKV) is a single-stranded RNA arbovirus (genus Alphavirus, family Togaviridae) that is transmitted to humans by the bite of infected mosquitoes [1]. It causes chikungunya fever (CHIKF), an illness characterized by the sudden onset of fever and severe arthralgia known to cause chronic morbidity. The virus rarely causes a fatal infection; however, it is known to cause great morbidity to those affected, sometimes extending from weeks to years. "Chikungunya" is a word taken from the Makonde language in Tanzania which means "that which bends up" and refers to the bent posture observed in patients secondary to the severe pain in their joints [2]. The disease was first identified in Tanzania in 1952 by RW Ross. After its discovery, outbreaks of chikungunya typically occurred in Asia and Africa. However, in 2004, the CHIKV reached India and several islands in the Indian Ocean, causing major outbreaks that affected more than 1 million people [3]. Since then, the virus has reached new regions, including the Americas and Europe.

The clinical picture of CHIKV and dengue virus are indistinguishable and accurate diagnosis of these infections on clinical grounds alone is somewhat challenging. It is believed that the CHIKV has been present on the African continent for centuries, from back when science was not capable of identifying it [4].

Three distinct CHIKV genotypes have been identified, based on their geographic distribution: West-African, East/Central/South African (ECSA), and Asian isolates. They are responsible for major epidemics around the world, and the identification of the virus by its corresponding genotype is achieved through gene sequencing [5].

During inter-epidemic periods, the CHIKV is conserved through an enzootic cycle in places where it is endemic (such as Africa and Asia) and an urban cycle when the virus reaches the cities. In the enzootic cycle, continuous transmission of the pathogen occurs between wild animals and vectors. Non-human primates (NHP) serve as the reservoir for the virus, and the mosquitoes from the *Aedes genus* are the vectors responsible for the transmission of the virus. It is known that the CHIKV can use animals such as buffalos, rodents, and birds as hosts, but the critical host for enzootic circulation is not known with certainty [6].

A spillover of the virus can occur when people who live in rural areas close to these virus reservoir cycles are bitten by an infected mosquito. If these people then travel to urban areas in which there are viable vectors, more people could almost certainly be infected. In urban areas, the virus is transmitted by mosquitoes of the *Aedes aegypti* and *Aedes albopictus* species. It is preserved and further spread in an autochthonous cycle in which continuous transmission occurs between mosquitoes and humans. In this type of transmission, infected mosquitoes transmit the virus to a person, enabling that individual to then contaminate the mosquitoes which feed on his or her blood, thus continuing the cycle [7].

The species *A. aegypti* was the principal vector involved in the outbreaks in Africa [8]. However, during the outbreaks in Asia, the territories of the Indian Ocean, Europe, and the Caribbean, *A. albopictus* was identified as the principal vector. This change in the species of the vector occurred because the virus acquired a new mutation which enhanced its ability to use *A. albopictus* as a vector. This mosquito species, originally from Southeast Asia, has shown a great ability to adapt to other climates, allowing it to spread into places that are non-endemic for the CHIKV [5, 9]. For this reason, the CHIKV is a latent threat for many countries, and thus new diagnostic and preventive measures are in need.

2. History

2.1 First sights

In 1952, the first CHIKV case was reported in the Makonde Plateaus region in Tanzania. The virus was isolated from the serum of several febrile patients and mosquitoes in 1953 by RW Ross [10]. Then in 1958, the first laboratory confirmed CHIKV outbreak in Asia was reported in Bangkok, Thailand [11]. Many countries in Southeast Asia, along with countries located in Central, Southern, and Western Africa continued to report sporadic outbreaks up to 1980. However, activity dwindled in the latter half of the 20th century.

2.2 Reemergence and increase dispersion of the chikungunya virus

For five decades, CHIKV was limited to sub-Saharan Africa and Southeast Asia. However, a new landscape developed at the beginning of the millennium. In 2004, an outbreak originated in Lamu Island on the coast of Kenya. Cases peaked in July, with an estimated 13,500 infected. In November, the disease reached Mombasa and the Comoros, resulting in a large outbreak that continued through 2005. It is estimated that 63% of the population may have been infected with CHIKV in Grande

Comore. This epidemic continued to spread to other islands in the Indian ocean in the following 2 years [12].

Between 2005 and 2007 the island of Reunion experienced an outbreak that affected 38.8% of its 785,000 inhabitants [13]. Unusual clinical manifestations were reported, including neurologic complications, increased mortality rate, and 41 cases of mother-to-child CHICKV transmission in the context of intrapartum maternal viremia. The cause of this phenomenon was found to be a single alanine-to-valine acquired mutation in the envelope protein E1 glycoprotein at position 226 (E1-A226V) of the ECSA genotype of the CHIKV. The mutation increased the virus infectivity of the island's native mosquitoes (*A. albopictus*). It led to greater and more effective dissemination of the disease due to the abundance of the arthropod vector [14]. Before the introduction of this mutation, the *A. aegypti* mosquito was the predominant vector used by the CHIKV. This mutation enabled the genotype to spread with a different vector, which is also present in other regions.

2.3 Asia

CHIKV has been circulating through Asia since the 1950s with sporadic outbreaks caused primarily by the Asian lineage. Significant expansion in its geographic distribution ensued from 2005 onwards. One of the countries with the highest disease burden was India. Between 2005 and 2006, the disease reemerged infecting 1.4 million individuals and dispersed to 17 of India's 28 providences [3]. The ECSA genotype was responsible for the outbreak, and *A. albopictus* was identified as the main vector in several areas. However, phylogenetic analysis indicates that this outbreak was due to a wild-type at E1–226, a different cluster to the La Reunion E1–226V lineage [15].

Other prominent outbreaks, caused by the ECSA lineage containing the E1–226 V mutation, were reported in Sri Lanka in 2006 (>36,000 cases), Malaysia in 2007, and in Thailand and Singapore in 2008–2009. In Cambodia, the first case of CHIKV was detected in 1961. The virus re-emerged in 2011 and a large outbreak occurred in the village of Trapeang Roka Kampong Speu Province in March 2012 [16].

The first imported sporadic case of the disease in China was described in Xishuangbanna, Yunnan Province, in 1987. The first documented community-based outbreak of CHIK fever was declared in the Xincun community of Wanjiang district in Dongguan city of Guangdong province on October 2010; 253 cases were recorded, of which 129 were laboratory confirmed. The outbreak was considered a local outbreak of CHIK fever caused by an imported case or vector, although the source is unclear [17].

According to the Indonesian Ministry of Health, chikungunya cases were initially reported in 1973 on Samarinda (Kalimantan island). The first virologically confirmed epidemic was reported in Jambi province of Sumatra island in June 1982. After a gap of approximately 20 years, the virus reappeared in Indonesia in 2001, causing outbreaks in 24 areas throughout Indonesia until 2004. Later, in 2009 and 2010, West and Central Indonesia were hit by the disease, causing 137,655 cases [18]. Studies suggest that the introduction of the ECSA genotype again is the culprit behind the massive outbreaks. After 2010, detected cases decreased dramatically. In 2011, CHIKV strains belonging to the Asian genotype and the ECSA genotype were circulating in different regions of Indonesia.

2.4 Europe

Since 2007, viremic travel-related cases have generated sporadic events of local CHIKV transmission throughout Europe. The first autochthonous outbreak was reported in the Emilia-Romagna region in north-eastern Italy in August 2007.

The virus was introduced by a traveler from South-West India who carried the ECSA strain. Sequencing demonstrated the presence of the E1–226 V mutation. Local transmission was facilitated by high levels of *A. albopictus* in Italy when the index patient arrived. More than 200 laboratory-confirmed cases were reported of which one person died: an 83-year-old man with underlying medical conditions. Vector control measures and drop in temperature associated to seasonal change interrupted CHIKV transmission [19, 20].

In France three outbreaks have occurred in the last 10 years. The first was in September 2010 in southern France. The initial source was a 7-year-old girl that had returned from Rajasthan, India. Two local children contracted the disease. In October 2014, a 12-case outbreak was detected in a district of Montpellier, a town in the south of France colonized by the arthropod vector *A. albopictus* since 2010 [21]. An individual returning from central Africa living in the affected district was identified as the primary case. Subsequently, in 2017, 17 cases distributed in two clusters were reported by French authorities: 11 cases in Le Cannet-des-Maures and 6 cases in Taradeau. The virus circulating in France belongs to an ECSA sub-lineage that includes isolates from the Central African region (e.g. Gabon, Republic of Congo) and carries an adaptive E1-A226V mutation [22].

An outbreak in the Italian regions of Lazio and Calabriin was also reported in the summer of 2017. Between the months of August to November, 270 cases of CHIKV were confirmed. This latest epidemic outnumbered the outbreak that occurred near the Adianic coast a decade earlier. The CHIKV strain isolated from humans and *A. albopictus* mosquitoes in Italy in 2017 showed a high similitude with virus strains ravaging in India and Pakistan at that time and did not carry the A226V mutation [23–25].

Other countries in Europe, such as Spain, Portugal, Germany, and Russia, have reported cases of CHIKV in travelers; however, no cases of native transmission have occurred thus far. As such, the frequency of travel enhances the risk of local transmission in *A. albopictus*-infested European regions, highlighting the potential to establish transmission cycles. Although a massive influx of travelers returning from the Americas where the Asian CHIKV genotype has caused around one million cases, no Asian genotype-related autochthonous transmission of CHIKV has been reported in Europe.

2.5 America and the Caribbean

The first sighting of CHIKV infection in the Western Hemisphere was in 2010 in Rio de Janeiro, Brazil in an area with high propensity for dengue infection due to predominance of the competent vector *A aegypti* [26]. The first autochthonous case of CHIKV was confirmed on December 2013 in the Collectivity of Saint Martin. The outbreak was thought to be caused by the frequent travel of residents between the islands of the Caribbean [27]. Subsequently, most territories in the Caribbean reported locally acquired CHIKF cases. By 2017, CHIKV infection had spread to 45 countries and territories in the Caribbean, North, Central and South America and over 2.5 million suspected cases and confirmed [28]. Dominican Republic (41%) and Suriname (90.4%) experienced attack rates comparable to those noted in Malaysia (55.6%) and India (37.5%). But are far higher than the attack rate observed in La Reunion (16.5%) [29].

The CHIKV found in the Caribbean corresponds to the Asian strain, and its principal vector is the *A. aegypti* mosquito [30, 31]. This genotype, which does not have the A226V mutation in the E1 gene, has been widely reported in both Central America and South America. The introduction of these strains into the Americas could result in a wider spread of the virus, because the *A. albopictus* mosquito is present in most of these regions [4].

Several months after the CHIKV arrived at the Caribbean, the state of Florida, in the United States, reported 11 autochthonous cases during the summer of 2014 [4]. During that year, 243 imported cases were reported in 31 states, Puerto Rico, and the US Virgin Islands [32].

There were 475 imported CHIKF cases reported in countries belonging to the European Union during the period of 2008 to 2012 [33]. Most of these imported cases matched the times when outbreaks were occurring in endemic countries. For this reason, the establishment of the CHIKV in the Caribbean poses a great threat to European countries due to the high number of travelers from the latter to the former. This implies that more diagnostic and surveillance measures need to be implemented in regions where the CHIKV could thrive, in order to prevent further outbreaks in new places and regions where the virus has not reached before [34].

2.6 Where are we today?

CHIKV outbreaks continue to appear thought the world. In 2020, a total of 27, 540 cases were reported in three provinces in continental Africa (District of Abéché, Biltine, and Abdi) [35]. The most affected age group are those 15 years and over. The majority of cases developed a high fever, headache, and joint pain. In America and the Caribbean, countries such as Colombia, Costa Rica, Ecuador, El Salvador, Mexico, Nicaragua, Paraguay, Peru and Venezuela have detected cases of CHICKV. In the United States, 21 CHIKV cases have been reported to the CDC from travelers returning from an affected area. No cases acquired through presumed local mosquito-borne transmission. According to the European Center for Disease Prevention and Control the countries with the most reported cases in the last year are Thailand, India and Brazil (**Figure 1**).

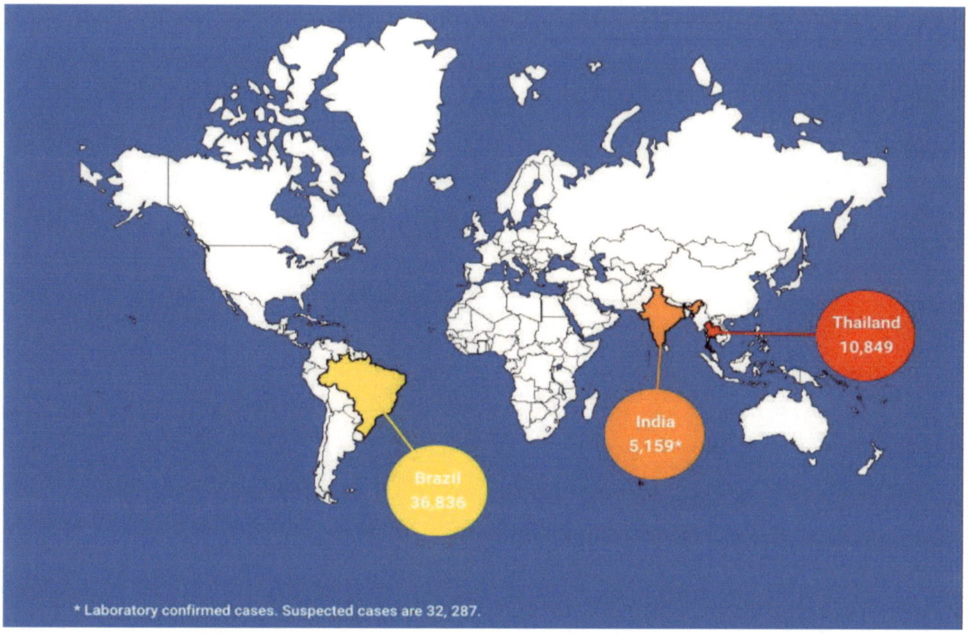

Figure 1.
Countries with the most reported CHIKV cases in 2020 according to the ECDC.

3. Conclusion

Once a local disease, CHIKV has spread to the majority of countries worldwide. Since its discovery in Tanzania in 1952, it has afflicted millions of people throughout tropical and sub-tropical regions. Individuals infected develop CHIKF characterized by severe polyarthralgia, headache, maculopapular rash, myalgia, and nausea/vomiting.

The first viremic wave took place between 1960 and 1980, affecting various regions in Africa and Southeast Asia. Evolution of the vector-borne RNA virus around 2005, lead to its dissemination into naïve areas such as America and Europe. Global expansion was also influenced by acquisition of a second competent vector *A. albopictus*, and travel of human carriers between affected and non-affected regions. As seen with the outbreaks in Europe, even temperate regions may experience severe outbreaks in the future.

CHIKV has become a global public health challenge. There are no current licensed vaccines and treatment strategies aim to relief symptoms. Therefore, re-emergence and spread to new places encourages further evaluation of the pathogenesis of this disease, in order to develop new preventive, diagnostic, and therapeutic options. For the time being, CHIKV outbreaks continue to be a threat and preparedness for the prevention and control of chikungunya outbreaks is key.

Acknowledgements

Giovanni F. Ramírez-Arroyo, M.D.

Conflict of interest

The authors declare no conflict of interest.

Appendices and nomenclature

CHIKF	chikungunya fever
CHIKV	chikungunya virus
ECDC	European Center for Disease Prevention and Control

Author details

Maria Zavala-Colon[1] and Juan A. Gonzalez-Sanchez[2]*

1 School of Medicine, Emergency Medicine Resident, University of Puerto Rico Medical Sciences Campus, San Juan, Puerto Rico

2 School of Medicine, Emergency Medicine Department, University of Puerto Rico Medical Sciences Campus, San Juan, Puerto Rico

*Address all correspondence to: juan.gonzalez30@upr.edu

References

[1] Tomasello D, Schlagenhauf P. Chikungunya and dengue auto chthonous cases in Europe, 2007-2012. Travel Med Infect Dis 2013;11:274-284.

[2] Lumsden WH. An epidemic of virus disease in Southern Province, Tanganyika Territory, in 1952-53. II. General description and epidemiology. Trans R Soc Trop Med Hyg 1955;49:33-57.

[3] Centers for Disease Control and Prevention and Panamerican Health Organization. Preparedness and Response for Chikungunya Virus Introduction in the Americas. Washington, DC: PAHO; 2011.

[4] Weaver SC, Forrester NL. Chikungunya: Evolutionary history and recent epidemic spread. Antiviral Res 2015;120:32-39.

[5] Lo Presti A, Lai A, Cella E, Zehender G, Ciccozzi M. Chikungunya virus, epidemiology, clinics and phylogenesis: A review. Asian Pac J Trop Med 2014;7:925-932.

[6] Kading RC, Borland EM, Cranfield M, Powers AM. Prevalence of antibodies to alphaviruses and flaviviruses in free-ranging game animals and non-human primates in the greater Congo basin. J Wildl Dis 2013;49:587-599.

[7] Staples JE, Breiman RF, Powers AM. Chikungunya fever: an epidemiological review of a re-emerging infectious disease. Clin Infect Dis 2009;49: 942-948.

[8] Diallo M, Thonnon J, Traore-Lamizana M, Fontenille D. Vectors of Chikungunya virus in Senegal: Current data and transmission cycles. Am J Trop Med Hyg 1999;60:281-286.

[9] Gratz NG. Critical review of the vector status of *Aedes albopictus*. Med Vet Entomol 2004;18:215-227.

[10] ROSS RW. The Newala epidemic. III. The virus: isolation, pathogenic properties and relationship to the epidemic. J Hyg (Lond). 1956;54(2):177-191. doi:10.1017/s0022172400044442

[11] Hammon WM, Rudnick A, Sather GE. Viruses associated with epidemic hemorrhagic fevers of the Philippines and Thailand. Science. 1960 Apr 15;131(3407):1102-3. doi: 10.1126/science.131.3407.1102. PMID: 14399343.

[12] Zeller H, Van Bortel W, Sudre B. Chikungunya: Its History in Africa and Asia and Its Spread to New Regions in 2013-2014. J Infect Dis. 2016 Dec 15;214(suppl 5):S436-S440. doi: 10.1093/infdis/jiw391. PMID: 27920169.

[13] Staikowsky F, Talarmin F, Grivard P, Souab A, Schuffenecker I, Le Roux K, et al. Prospective study of chikungunya virus acute infection in the Island of La Réunion during the 2005-2006 outbreak. PLoS One. 2009;4:1-9

[14] Tsetsarkin KA, Vanlandingham DL, McGee CE, Higgs S. A single mutation in Chikungunya virus affects vector specificity and epidemic potential. PLoS Pathog 2007;3:1895-1906.

[15] Rojjanaporn Pulmanausahakul, Sittiruk Roytrakul, Prasert Auewarakul, Duncan R. Smith, Chikungunya in Southeast Asia: understanding the emergence and finding solutions, International Journal of Infectious Diseases, Volume 15, Issue 10, 2011, pages e671-e676.

[16] Braira Wahid, Amjad Ali, Shazia Rafique, Muhammad Idrees, Global expansion of chikungunya virus: mapping the 64-year history, International Journal of Infectious Diseases, Volume 58, 2017, Pages 69-76, ISSN 1201-9712.

[17] Qiaoli, Z., Jianfeng, H., De, W., Zijun, W., Xinguang, Z., Haojie, Z., Fan,

D., Zhiquan, L., Shiwen, W., Zhenyu, H., Yonghui, Z., Changwen, K., Dakang, Y., Wenjia, L., Deqiong, L., & Pinghua, C. (2012). Maiden outbreak of chikungunya in Dongguan city, Guangdong province, China: epidemiological characteristics. PloS one, 7(8), e42830. https://doi.org/10.1371/journal.pone.0042830.

[18] Harapan, H., Michie, A., Mudatsir, M., Nusa, R., Yohan, B., Wagner, A. L., Sasmono, R. T., & Imrie, A. (2019). Chikungunya virus infection in Indonesia: a systematic review and evolutionary analysis. BMC infectious diseases, 19(1), 243. https://doi.org/10.1186/s12879-019-3857-y

[19] Amraoui F, Failloux AB. Chikungunya: an unexpected emergence in Europe. Curr Opin Virol. 2016 Dec;21:146-150. doi: 10.1016/j.coviro.2016.09.014. Epub 2016 Oct 20. PMID: 27771517.

[20] Watson R. (2007). Europe witnesses first local transmission of chikungunya fever in Italy. BMJ (Clinical research ed.), 335(7619), 532-533. https://doi.org/10.1136/bmj.39332.708738.DB

[21] Delisle E, Rousseau C, Broche B, Leparc-Goffart I, L'Ambert G, Cochet A, Prat C, Foulongne V, Ferre JB, Catelinois O, Flusin O, Tchernonog E, Moussion IE, Wiegandt A, Septfons A, Mendy A, Moyano MB, Laporte L, Maurel J, Jourdain F, Reynes J, Paty MC, Golliot F. Chikungunya outbreak in Montpellier, France, September to October 2014. Euro Surveill. 2015 Apr 30;20(17):21108. doi: 10.2807/1560-7917.es2015.20.17.21108. PMID: 25955774.

[22] European Centre for Disease Prevention and Control. Clusters of autochthonous chikungunya cases in Italy, first update – 9 October 2017. Stockholm: ECDC; 2017.

[23] Lindh E, Argentini C, Remoli ME, Fortuna C, Faggioni G, Benedetti E, et al. The Italian 2017 Outbreak Chikungunya Virus Belongs to an Emerging *Aedes albopictus*-Adapted Virus Cluster Introduced From the Indian Subcontinent. Open Forum Infect Dis. 2019 Jan;6(1):ofy321.

[24] Riccardo F, Di Luca M, Venturi G, Del Manso M. A secondary autochthonous Chikungunya outbreak in a village in Calabria, Italy. Provisionally accepted, under review. Emerging Infectious Diseases 2019.

[25] Riccardo, F., Venturi, G., Di Luca, M., Del Manso, M., Severini, F., Andrianou, X, Rizzo, C. (2019). Secondary Autochthonous Outbreak of Chikungunya, Southern Italy, 2017. Emerging Infectious Diseases, 25(11), 2093-2095. https://dx.doi.org/10.3201/eid2511.180949.

[26] Albuquerque IG, Marandino R, Mendonça AP, et al. Chikungunya virus infection: report of the first case diagnosed in Rio de Janeiro, Brazil. Rev Soc Bras Med Trop. 2012;45(1):128-129.

[27] Van Bortel W, Dorleans F, Rosine J, Blateau A, Rousset D, Matheus S, et al. Chikungunya outbreak in the Caribbean region, December 2013 to March 2014, and the significance for Europe. Euro Surveill. 2014;19. pii: 20759.

[28] Chikungunya virus. Cumulative Case Report. [PAHO Web site]. December 2020. Available from: https://www.paho.org/data/index.php/en/mnu-topics/chikv-en/550-chikv-weekly-en.html. [Accessed: December 2020].

[29] Wimalasiri-Yapa, B., Stassen, L., Huang, X., Hafner, L. M., Hu, W., Devine, G. J., Yakob, L., Jansen, C. C., Faddy, H. M., Viennet, E., & Frentiu, F. D. (2019). Chikungunya virus in Asia – Pacific: a systematic review. Emerging microbes & infections, 8(1), 70-79. https://doi.org/10.1080/22221751.2018. 1559708

[30] Leparc-Goffart I, Nougairede A, Cassadou S, Prat C, de Lamballerie X. Chikungunya in the Americas. Lancet 2014;383:514.

[31] Ben-Chetrit E, Schwartz E. Vector-borne diseases in Haiti: A review. Travel Med Infect Dis 2015;13:150-158.

[32] Lara HH, Sepulveda-de Leon VH, Mureyko L, Ixtepan-Turrent L. Chikungunya in the United States. J Hum Virol Retrovirology. 2014;1:00015.

[33] De Valk H, Leparc-Goffart I, Paty M, Reusken C, van den Kerkho H, Braks M. Rapid risk assessment: Autochthonous cases of chikungunya fever on the Caribbean island, Saint Martin. ECDC Rapid Risk Assess 2013. Available at: Url: https://ecdc.europa.eu/en/publications-data/rapid-risk-assessment-autochthonous-cases-chikungunya-fever-caribbean-island. Accessed July 15, 2016.

[34] Johansson MA. Chikungunya on the move. Trends Parasitol 2015;31: 43-45.

[35] Chikungunya Virus. Center for Disease Control and Prevention. [CDC Web site]. November 2020. Available from: https://www.cdc.gov/chikungunya/geo/index.html. [Accessed: December 2020].

Section 3

Epidemiology

Chapter 3

Epidemiology of Chikungunya in Indonesia

Tri Baskoro Tunggul Satoto and Nur Alvira Pascawati

Abstract

Chikungunya is a zoonotic disease which is caused by the Chikungunya virus (CHIKV) and transmitted by infected *Aedes spp* mosquito. In Indonesia, CHIKV is a re-emerging disease, which means that it is a disease that has gone for a long time, but then it spreads again and causes outbreaks frequently. CHIKV presence in Indonesia was first reported in 1979 in Bengkulu City causing substantial acute and chronic morbidity. After disappearing for 16 years, the CHIKV outbreak spreaded again in 24 regions throughout Indonesia from 2001 to 2003. In 2009 and 2010, CHIKV outbreaks hit western and central regions of Indonesia and increased from 3,000 cases per year to 83,000 and 52,000 cases per year. The burden of this disease is unclear due to insufficient monitoring and diagnosis. The spread and transmission of CHIKV in Indonesia is very high, due to travel, competent vectors, and the vulnerability of the population. In addition, the evolution of viruses, globalization and climate change has accelerated the spread of this virus. Effective antiviral treatment and vaccines do not yet exist, so early detection and appropriate management can help reducing the burden of this disease. Monitoring and risk assessment to reduce human-vector contact are also needed to reduce the impact of chikungunya.

Keywords: Indonesia, CHIKV, re-emerging disease, epidemiology

1. Introduction

Chikungunya is a zoonotic disease caused by the Chikungunya virus (CHIKV), and transmitted by infected *Aedes spp* mosquito. CHIKV is an important but often overlooked cause of fever in the tropics and subtropics [1, 2]. The disease is of little interest in the medical community and causes less fear when compared to other arboviruses such as DENV. The reappearance of CHIKV after a long absence has only recently attracted global attention because of its explosive attack, rapid spread, high morbidity, and various clinical manifestations [3–6]. However, the diagnosis of CHIKV is still very low due to overlapping clinical presentation with DENV and other endemic infections [7] as well as the lack of capacity for CHIKV testing [8]. Viral evolution, globalization, and climate change can further accelerate the spread of CHIKV, whereas specific antiviral treatments and effective vaccines do not yet exist [9].

In Indonesia, CHIKV is a re-emerging disease, which means that it is a disease that has gone for a long time, but it then spreads again [10]. Evidence from historical reports indicates that the first spread of CHIKV occurred in 1779 in Jakarta, but at that time the disease was referred to as kidinga pepo [11, 12]. This is widely recognized by arbovirus experts as the first report on chikungunya in Indonesia, although it cannot be proven by molecular analysis [13]. Virologically confirmed chikungunya outbreaks were first reported in June 1982 in Jambi province on the island of Sumatra, followed by outbreaks between 1983 and 1984 [14]. CHIKV was no longer recorded in Indonesia for about 20 years, before the infection re-emerged and caused several outbreaks in South Sumatra, Aceh and West Java in early 2001 [15]. In 2009 and 2010, CHIKV outbreaks hit western and central region of Indonesia started from approximately 3,000 cases per year increased to 83,000 and 52,000 cases per year [15–26]. After 2010, detected cases fell to 3,000 per year. Except during outbreaks, the number of cases are likely to be underestimated because diagnosis is often based solely on clinical presentation [27, 28].

2. Epidemiology

Arboviruses are viruses that undergo a cycle of transmission between a blood-eating arthropod vector and reinforcing vertebrate host. Mosquitoes are the main vector of arbovirus transmission and human involvement in the transmission cycle is incidental [29]. It is estimated that 3.9 billion people in 120 countries are at risk of being infected with one of the three main arboviruses, namely: namely CHIKV, Dengue virus (DENV) and Zika virus (ZIKV) [30]. An outbreak of chikungunya with specific features was first reported in the Southern province of Tanzania's Tanganyika region in 1952 [31, 32]. Later sporadic outbreaks of chikungunya were identified in parts of Africa and Asia during the 1950s and 1960s, followed by a clear comeback in the 2000s [33]. Since 2005, large-scale outbreaks of chikungunya have hit the southwest Indian Ocean and Southeast Asia [34–43]. In La Réunion, the outbreak affected about a third of the population [35, 44], and in India the virus infected more than 1.3 million people during 2005–2006 [45] and CHIKV then spread to Southeast Asia including Indonesia.

3. Definition

The diseases caused by CHIKV are clinically difficult to distinguish and accurately diagnose from diseases caused by DENV solely on clinical symptomps [46, 47]. Although previous literature has shown that, the proportion of symptoms in people infected with CHIKV is higher than DENV [48], however a systematic review shows that asymptomatic chikungunya has very wide variability with a percentage of around 3,2% during 2005–2006 in La Réunion to 82,1% during 2012–2013 in Philippines [49]. The definition includes four categories of cases: (1). Clinical case of acute, characterized with fever (temperature above 38.5° C/101.3° F]) and arthritis or joint pain (sometimes disabling) with epidemiological criteria and/or acute onset and laboratory criteria; (2). Atypical case, characterized with laboratory confirmed clinical cases accompanied with other manifestations (ie, cardiovascula, neurological, ophthalmological, dermatological, hepatic, renal, respiratory, or conditions of hematological); (3). Cases of severe acute, characterized with laboratory-confirmed clinical cases of CHIKV with life-threatening abnormal function of minimal 1 organ or system and requiring inpatient; (4). Chronic cases of suspected/confirmed, characterized with a previous clinical diagnosis of chikungunya 12 weeks after onset of symptoms and indicating at least 1 rheumatological manifestation (ie, edema, stiffness, or pain) that was persistent or recurring [50].

The highest CHIKV genotype in Asia has been noted to be asymptomatic found in Philippines with a percentage of 82.1% [51]. Common symptoms of chikungunya include high fever, severe joint and muscle pain, rash, photophobia and headache [52, 53]. Severe symptoms implicated vital organs may develop during infection, like encephalitis [54, 55], myelopathy, myelitis [55], encephalopathy [55–57], neuroretinitis [58], optic neuropathy and Guillain's Syndrome [55, 58]. Barré [55, 58], myocarditis [57], hepatitis [59], acute interstitial nephritis [60], severe sepsis, septic shock [61] and multi-organ failure [57–59, 62, 63]. In rare cases, infection can be fatal [44, 59–61, 63]. Perinatal CHIKV infection can cause symptoms such as microcephaly and cerebral palsy [64]. In adults with persistent arthralgia/arthritis, alopecia and depression are the other symptoms most frequently noted [65–67]. A meta-analysis found that about 25% of chikungunya cases caused chronic inflammatory rheumatism and 14% had chronic arthritis [68].

4. Incidence and mortality

Eleven annual reports from the Indonesian Ministry of Health (MoH) were identified between 2004 and 2019 [15, 17–26]. These data show that the lowest incidence rate of CHIKV occurred in 2005 with 0.16/100,000 person-years [15] while the highest incidence rate was recorded in 2009 to 36.2 cases per 100,000 person-years [23]. In 2009, more than 83 thousand cases CHIKV in Indonesia was reported circulating in 17 of 34 provinces (50%) [23]. Cases began to decline in 2010 with 52,703 cases and continued to decline significantly until 2018, but again increased in 2019 with an incidence of 5,042 cases (**Figure 1**), but some districts did not report cases of chikungunya [69]. Based on a report from the MoH, this increase was due to relatively humid weather conditions with high rainfall, long periods of rain and immunity in areas that had been affected [69].

The case map by province showed that the CHIKV was not evenly distributed across Indonesia. The highest incidence of chikungunya occurred in Sumatra, Kalimantan and Java. However, Papua and West Papua provinces of Indonesia did not report chikungunya in 2008 and 2016. The shift in cases in several Indonesian provinces in 2019 has changed with the highest cases in West Java, Lampung and Gorontalo.

CHIKV cases that occurred in Indonesia during the 26 years period (1989–2014) actually originated from several countries. During that period there were 195 cases of chikungunya reported from travelers returning from Australia (128 cases) [70–77] Taiwan (47 cases) [47, 78–79], Japan (4 cases) [80–81] and other countries.

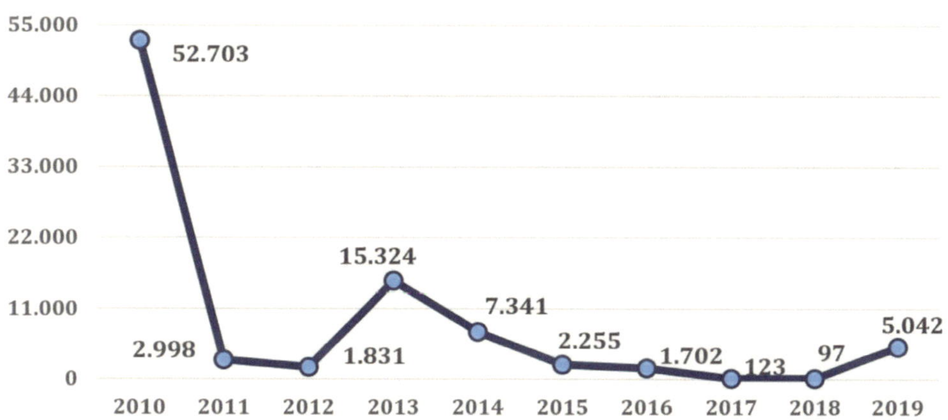

Figure 1.
Trend and number of chikungunya cases based on the Ministry of Health report of the Republic of Indonesia from 2010 to 2019.

in Asia, Europe and the Pacific (16 cases) [82–88]. Based on the results of investigations on five outbreaks that occurred, there were no reports of deaths due to chikungunya [40, 45, 64, 89, 90]. In addition, in eleven annual reports from the Indonesian MoH, for 44 years (1973 to 2016) there were also no deaths related to CHIKV infection [39, 41, 42, 44, 46–49, 51].

5. CHIKV genotype circulating in Indonesia

Sixteen studies that reported on the CHIKV genotype identified circulating in Indonesia were 130 viral sequences [27, 38, 47, 78, 79, 82, 87, 88, 91–98]. There were seven studies conducted on local populations [27, 28, 38, 91, 93, 96, 98] and eight studies with viruses isolated from travelers returning from Indonesia [47, 78, 79, 83, 87, 88, 92, 97]. One study did not specify whether the virus was isolated in local residents or in travelers [82]. Of the seven studies, four were conducted in non-outbreak conditions [27, 28, 93, 96], two investigations were carried out during an outbreak of chikungunya [38, 91] and one study did not specify the condition [99]. Most of the viruses isolated from travelers originated in Taiwan [47, 78, 79]. Another virus was collected from travelers returning from Singapore [92], France [97], the Netherlands [82], Russia [83], and Germany [88]. Most of the CHIKV isolated from Indonesia belonged to the Asian genotype and partially from the ECSA genotype. Of these ECSA viruses, two were isolated from local residents in 2011 [38] and eight others were isolated from travelers returning from Indonesia between 2008 and 2010 [47, 87, 92]. The ESCA virus sample during the 2008–2011 period in Indonesia was included in the Indian Ocean Lineage (IOL) because in the same period it was also circulating in Southeast Asian countries such as China, South Korea, Malaysia, Sri Lanka, Thailand, Singapore, and Myanmar [93].

6. Vectors of CHIKV

The vector that plays a role in CHIKV and DENV is the *Aedes aegypti* mosquito and the potential vector is the *Aedes albopictus* mosquito (The Asian Tiger Mosquito) [25]. The *Aedes* mosquito is a mosquito that belongs to the Diptera order and has more than 950 species [100]. Transmission of the disease caused by the *Aedes* mosquito can manifest itself in humans and animals. The *Aedes* mosquito usually lives in temperate and tropical climates. However, due to the current uncertain climate change, this mosquito is able to expand its habitat [100]. The following is an explanation of the mosquito that transmits CHIKV:

6.1 Taxonomy

Kingdom: Animalia.
Phylum: Arthropoda.
Class: Insecta.
Order: Diptera.
Family: Culicidae.
Subfamily: Culicinae.
Tribes: Aedini.
Genus: Aedes.
Species: Aedes aegypti and Aedes albopictus.

6.2 Morphology

6.2.1 Adult Aedes aegypti *Mosquito*

The *Aedes aegypti* mosquito was first discovered in Southeast Asia and was identified in Malaysia and Thailand in the early 20th century. Apart from carrying CHIKV, these mosquitoes are also carriers of yellow fever and dengue fever. The body of the *Aedes aegypti* mosquito consists of the head, thorax and abdomen. On the head area there is a proboscis, antenna, maxillary palpus, and clype. On the thorax area there is the scutum, and at the end of the thorax is the scutellum. Proboscis in males is longer (0.76 ± 0.04 mm) than in females (0.53 ± 0.06 mm) but only in females the structure is formed to suck blood while males only suck nectar. The antennae in males are longer (0.57 ± 0.03 mm) and also have denser hair than females (0.52 ± 0.07 mm) [101–103]. Specific Characteristic of the adult mosquito *Aedes aegypti* is the scutum on the thorax is black or brown with a pair of submedian-longitudinal white stripes, but without median-longitudinal white stripes, or with white lute-shaped markings. Mesepimeron with two nicely separated white scale patches. The anterior part of the midfemur with longitudinal white stripes, and the head of the clypeus with white scales. In addition, paratergite with wide white scales and palpomeric heads 4 with white scales on apex [102, 104].

6.2.2 Adult mosquito Aedes albopictus

Aedes albopictus is a type of mosquito that is currently the main vector in various parts of the world. Moreover, these mosquitoes have the ability to transmit various diseases (acting as vectors) from arbovirus to worms such as *Dirofilaria immitis* and vector for 22 arboviruses [105]. *Aedes albopictus* is medium in size (2–10 mm) and the males are smaller than the females. The males can also be distinguished by their more feathered antennae than the females [106]. Its abdomen area is covered by black scales. The morphological characteristics of *Aedes albopictus* are slightly different from *Aedes aegypti*. Scutum thorax of this species is characterized with a narrow median-longitudinal white stripe. Mesepimeron with inseparable white scaly patches, forming a white V-shaped patch. The anterior part of the midfemur has longitudinal white stripes and the head of the clypeus without white scales [102].

6.2.3 Eggs

Female *Aedes* mosquitoes usually lay eggs on a substrate that is on the surface of the water either in artificial or natural water containers [107]. *Aedes* eggs are white and soft when laid but later turn black and become hard and increase in size [108, 109]. Eggs of *Aedes aegypti* and *Aedes albopictus* do not form groups, but individually and float on the surface of a wet substrate such as water [110, 111]. *Aedes* eggs can survive dry conditions for months or years [110] and also these eggs can have viability despite being faced with excessive water conditions [112–114]. *Aedes* eggs can withstand extreme conditions because they have a shell or what is called an eggshell that protects the oocyte, egg, embryo from extreme conditions but is still able to exchange enough gas to survive [107]. The difference between *Aedes albopictus* and *Aedes aegypti* lies in the difference of the micropylar collar shape, where *Aedes aegypti*'s eggs have a prominent micropylar collar and in *Aedes albopictus* it is not too striking. *Aedes albopictus* has a large tubercle in the middle so it looks like a smoother, lighter one than in *Aedes aegypti*.

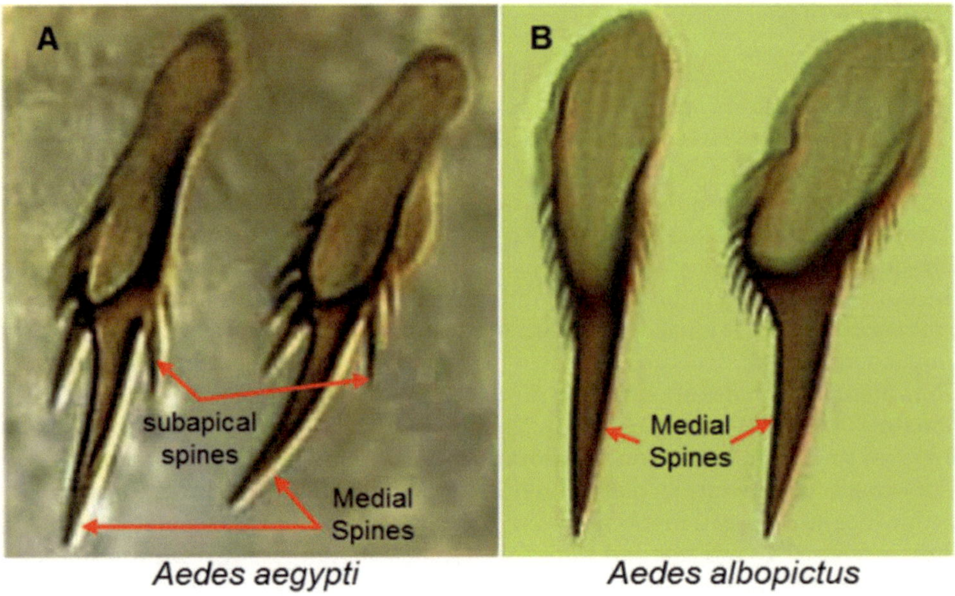

Figure 2.
The differences of comb scale on A. aegypti *dan* A. albopictus *[103, 104].*

6.2.4 Larvae

Aedes aegypti's larvae usually have an oval head, a thorax and also an abdomen consisting of 9 segments. On the posterior side, there are 4 lobes and also a siphon which functions to help breathing on the water surface. On the surface of the water, *Aedes* larvae will have a hanging position almost forming a vertical direction [102]. *Aedes aegypti* has a specific characteristic that its 8th abdominal segment has comb scales equipped with lateral spines (**Figure 2A**). Furthermore, *Aedes aegypti* larvae also has pectent teeth on the siphon. In addition, *Aedes aegypti* larvae has 5 pairs of hairs on its ventral brush. In *Aedes albopictus* mosquito larvae, the brush scales do not have lateral spines, pecten teeth with two branches while the ventral brush has 4 unpaired hairs (**Figure 2B**).

The life cycle of the *Aedes albopictus* mosquito is highly dependent on ambient temperature and pH of 5.2-7.6 with an optimal pH of about 6.8 and 7.6 in Asia [115]. Research conducted by Satoto, et al. States that the larvae of *Aedes aegypti* and *Aedes albopictus* can be found as much as 61% in flower pots, 15.38% bathtubs, containers, large and small buckets containing 55% water. *Aedes albopictus* larvae are active feeders, which means that they eat various kinds of organic matter in the water.

6.3 Bionomics

6.3.1 Breeding places

The breeding places habitats of the two vectors are somewhat different. For *Aedes aegypti*, its preferred place to lay eggs is in a clear water reservoir in the house, which is protected from the sun. Water reservoirs that can hold water for a long time make this habitat easy to breed [116, 117], such as bathtubs in bathrooms (toilets), bathtubs, drinking water reservoirs, buckets, jars, drums, and the like [101, 104, 118]. In Dar es Salaam, it is found in piped water systems due to intermittent water supply and rainwater storage which is used for community needs [119].

Aedes albopictus prefers to lay eggs in water reservoirs outside the house such as cans, bottles, discarded tires, tree holes, plant grooves, pieces of bamboo, and open coconuts. This shelter is not used for daily household needs. This is in accordance with the nature of *Aedes aegypti* which has a tendency as a house mosquito and *Aedes albopictus* which is an outdoor mosquito [100, 103, 117].

6.3.2 Feeding habit

The *Aedes aegypti* mosquito is anthropophagic, which means that it prefers to suck human blood in a single gonotrophic cycle [120]. While the *Aedes albopictus* mosquito is a more zoophagic, random bloodsucker [121], it has also been shown to exhibit strong anthropophagic behavior like *Aedes aegypti* [122]. To find their host, mosquitoes are active in the morning, which is around 8 am–10 am and in the afternoon 3 pm–5 pm [123]. Three days after sucking blood, female mosquitoes produce 100–200 eggs depending on the amount of blood sucked. The more blood it sucked, the more eggs will be produced [124].

6.3.3 Resting places

Places that mosquitoes prefer to rest while waiting to lay eggs are the ones which are dark, humidwith little wind [125]. *Aedes aegypti* prefers dark, damp, and hidden places in the house or building as a place to rest, including in the bedroom, in the bathroom, and in the kitchen. Indoors, a mosquito's preferred resting surface is under the furniture, hanging objects such as clothes and curtains, and walls. These mosquitoes are rarely found outdoors, in plants, or other protected areas. Meanwhile, the *Aedes albopictus* mosquito, known as the Asian tiger mosquito, prefers places outside the house, such as in tree holes, plant grooves, and gardens or forest edge areas [118, 126, 127].

6.3.4 Flight range

The movement of *Aedes aegypti* mosquitoes from breeding places to prey and rest areas is determined by the ability of mosquitoes to fly. The average flight range of the *Aedes aegypti* mosquito is about 100 m, but in certain circumstances these mosquitoes can fly up to several kilometers in an attempt to find breeding places to lay their eggs. The mosquito *Aedes albopictus* has a flight range of 400-600 m [128].

Several studies have shown that the average mosquito has a flight range (mainly related to migration) between 50 m and 50 km [129]. *Aedes albopictus*, a type of mosquito that breeds in containers, is a very weak flyer (mean maximum 676 m) [130]. The flight ability of mosquitoes is highly dependent on wind assistance as some species can disperse during periods of high winds and energy required to travel great distances. For active flight *Aedes aegypti* and *Aedes albopictus* depend on carbohydrates [131].

7. Prognosis

A retrospective study of 107 serologically proven cases of chikungunya infection (CHIKV) was conducted. All respondents had contracted the disease at least 3 years before; 87.9% had fully recovered, 3.7% had only occasional stiffness or mild discomfort, 2.8% had residual joint stiffness but no pain, while 5.6% had persistent pain and stiffness and frequent effusions. All patients with persistent joint pain and stiffness had very high antibody titres against the CHIK virus [132]. In some isolation, CHIKV performed in severe cases showed bleeding manifestations, neurological abnormalities, and heart muscle abnormalities. Sports activities can worsen clinical symptoms such as joint pain, especially in the morning. The knee joint can swell as can the wrist and finger joints [133]. CHIKV infection, both clinical and silent, will provide lifelong immunity, so it is difficult for the same disease to attack the same patient [134]. Most patients recover completely from infection, but in some cases, joint pain can last for months, or even years [135].

8. Incubation period and treatment based on the natural course of the disease

8.1 Incubation period

The incubation period occurs when the mosquito acquires the virus from the viremic host. After an average extrinsic incubation of 10 days, the mosquitoes can then transmit the virus to a host, such as humans. In humans bitten by infected mosquitoes, disease symptoms usually appear after an intrinsic mean incubation period of three to seven days (range: 1–12 days) [115].

8.2 Acute and chronic

Symptomatic or supportive treatment, consisting of rest and use of acetaminophen or paracetamol to relieve fever, and ibuprofen, naproxen, or other non-steroidal anti-inflammatory agents (NSAIDs) to relieve the rheumatic component of the disease. In patients with severe joint pain that does not resolve with NSAIDs, narcotics (e.g. morphine) or short-term corticosteroids may be used after evaluating the risk–benefit of these treatments. Patients are advised to drink plenty of fluids to replace fluids lost through sweating, vomiting, and other involuntary fluid losses [136].

8.3 Sub-acute and chronic

Recovery from CHIK will be a fairly long process (sometimes up to a year or even more) and persistent joint pain may require pain management, including long-term anti-inflammatory therapy. Although studies have shown that chloroquine phosphate provides some benefit [137], randomized, double-blind placebo-controlled trials have shown that it is not useful for treating joint symptoms [138]. Apart from pharmacotherapy, cases of prolonged arthralgia and joint stiffness can be treated with a gradual physiotherapy program [136].

8.4 Isolation

To prevent transmission to other people in the household, community, or hospital, sufferers of acute chikungunya (CHIKV) should avoid being bitten by the *Aedes aegypti* or *Aedes albopictus* mosquitoes during the viremic phase, which is usually the first week of illness. In addition, doctors or health workers visiting patients infected with CHIKV at home must also be careful not to be bitten by mosquitoes by wearing repellents and wearing long sleeves and pants [136]. One hospital-related CHIK infection has been identified in a healthcare provider due to the accidental needle puncture of a CHIK patient [139]. Some laboratory personnel also contracted CHIKV infection after handling infected blood [140]. This exposure indicates that direct contact transmission can occur.

9. Surveillance of chikungunya

Epidemiological surveillance is the key to detecting cases in a timely manner and a prompt and appropriate response is required with the active participation of all stakeholders. Surveillance activities are carried out to determine whether chikungunya (CHIKV) has entered an area, track the disease that has entered and follow it on an ongoing basis. The forms of CHIKV surveillance activities in Indonesia are: [136, 141].

9.1 Case definition

The case definition of CHIKV used in the surveillance system in Indonesia has been published in the Ministry of Health's National Guidelines for Chikungunya Prevention and Control followed World Health Organization (WHO) criteria [141]. In short, chikungunya cases are classified into three categories, namely: (1). Possible cases, diagnosed on clinical criteria alone as acute fever>38.5° C and severe arthralgia/arthritis which could not be explained by other medical conditions; (2). Probable cases, diagnosed based on clinical criteria as stated and epidemiological criteria (living or visiting epidemic areas); (3). Confirmed cases, diagnosed according to laboratory criteria that showed a positive result for viral isolation, RT-PCR, IgM antibody or a fourfold increase in IgG antibody.

9.2 Preparation phase

Strengthen the fever syndromic surveillance sentinel site, so that officers can detect cases of chikungunya (CHIKV). The percentage of patients presenting with fever and arthralgia or fever and arthritis with no known etiology (eg, testing negative for malaria or dengue), should be tested for CHIK in an adequate national referral laboratory [141].

9.3 Response phase

Once a case of chikungunya (CHIKV) is detected, an in-depth epidemiological investigation will be carried out to (1). Track the spread of viruses; (2). Monitor the possibility that cases have entered the surrounding area; (3). Describe the epidemiological features and main clinical features; (4). Assess the severity and impact on society; (5). Identify risk factors or factors that cause disease severity; (6) identify the circulating CHIKV lineage. These efforts will form the basis to develop effective control measures [136, 141].

9.4 Continuous transmission

Continuous surveillance to monitor changes in the epidemiology and ecology of CHIKV transmission. Any changes in surveillance at the national level should be communicated immediately to surveillance partners and other prevention units to ensure quality and uniformity of data collected [136, 141].

10. Vector surveillance and control

There are no specific antiviral treatments and vaccines that are effective yet, so the only method available to prevent infection is the reduction of human-vector contact [142]. We have done research about distribution of CHIKV vector transmission in Indonesia by taking locations that represent urban and rural areas, coastal and inland areas. The results of this study show on *Aedes aegypti* or *Aedes albopictus* or both were found in all sampling locations except in Warsadim, West Papua. Apart from Warsadim, there is only one site that does not have *Aedes aegypti*, namely Bugel in Yogyakarta Province, while 26 locations are free of *Aedes albopictus* [143]. Efforts to reduce CHIKV risk are carried out through an integrated vector management program component, including the following activities:

10.1 Vector monitoring and identification of high-risk areas

Retrospective analysis of dengue virus transmission in previous years can be carried out in the planning stage of chikungunya (CHIKV) to show areas where CHIKV is expected to circulate (given the similarities in the transmission cycle of this virus). Areas can be grouped in levels of risk of transmission, so they can be used to assign resources and priorities. For example, controlling or preventing transmission of CHIKV in the environment has resulted in many cases of dengue fever, thereby inhibiting viral amplification and spreading the virus to the immediate environment [144].

Programs should be able to systematically collect surveillance data for the vector density of *Aedes aegypti* and *Aedes albopictus*. The surveillance methods for *Aedes aegypti* and *Aedes albopictus* are quite varied and include a variety of methods to monitor egg production, larval location and density, pupa density, and adult mosquito density. This measure is used to asses the risk of outbreaks and to determine the appropriate vector control interventions [143]. Metodhs and tools, calculations and risk analysis with this measure have been widely discussed in the Dengue Hemorrhagic Fever guideline.

10.2 Self protection

Each individual can reduce the likelihood of transmission by using personal mosquito repellents. Babies and pregnant women who sleep or rest during the day should use a mosquito net. The use of insecticide-treated bed nets has the added benefit of killing mosquitoes that come into contact with the nets, thereby reducing vector-human contact with other household members. There are many insecticide products that can be used to treat mosquito nets safely or to make them last longer [136, 141, 142].

10.3 Prevention at the household and community level

The use of screened ventilation, or insulated windows and doors will reduce the entry of vectors into the house. Reducing and replacing containers that hold water over a long period of time can reduce vector breeding grounds [100, 104]. The number of adult mosquitoes in the home can be reduced by using commercially available aerosol sprays with pyrethroids and other household products, such as mosquito coils and electronics [145].

Prevention in community settings for CHIKV should be based on methods developed for dengue fever control to reduce vector mosquito density [146]. Dengue fever control programs that are carried out optimally will reduce the possibility of humans being infected when they come to an area that has the potential to cause secondary transmission and the formation of the virus. Dengue fever programs to control *Aedes* species that focus on larval control, often involving communities in environmental management and reduction of mosquito breeding sites [147].

However, community involvement has not been comprehensively incorporated into integrated vector management programs [147, 148].

11. Conclusion

The spread and transmission of CHIKV in Indonesia is very high due to its travel, competent vectors (the same vector as dengue fever), and the vulnerability of the population. Furthermore, the evolution of viruses, globalization and climate change has accelerated the spread of this virus. Timely case detection and prompt and appropriate response with active participation of all stakeholders are necessary to minimize cases of import and transmission that are increasingly widespread in Indonesia. The absence of treatments and effective vaccines makes the correct method for preventing infection is the reduction of human-vector contact through integrated vector management. Each of the discussions in this chapter can be used to improve early warning systems for detecting outbreaks, conducting epidemiological investigations, and preventing the spread of CHIKV.

Author details

Tri Baskoro Tunggul Satoto[1] and Nur Alvira Pascawati[2]*

1 Department of Parasitology, Faculty of Medicine, Gadjah Mada University, Indonesia

2 Public Health Study Program, Faculty of Health Science, Respati University of Yogyakarta, Indonesia

*Address all correspondence to: irha011185@yahoo.com; alvirapascawati@gmail.com

References

[1] Coffey L, Failloux AB, Weaver S: Chikungunya virus–vector interactions. Viruses. 2014: 6:11:4628-4663. DOI: 10.3390/v6114628. PMID: 25421891.

[2] Rezza G, El-Sawaf G, Faggioni G, Vescio F, Al Ameri R, De Santis R, et al: Co-circulation of dengue and chikungunya viruses, Al Hudaydah, Yemen, 2012. Emerg Infect Dis. 2014: 20:8:1351-1354. DOI: 10.3201/eid2008.131615. PMID: 25061762.

[3] Mohan A. Chikungunya fever strikes in Andhra Pradesh. Natl Med J India. 2006:19:24: 417-474.

[4] Simon F, Savini H, Parola P: Chikungunya: a paradigm of emergence and globalization of vector-borne diseases. Med Clin North Am. 2008:92:6:1323-1343. Doi: 10.1016/j.mcna.2008.07.008. PMID: 19061754.

[5] Chevillon C, Briant L, Renaud F, Devaux C: The Chikungunya threat: an ecological and evolutionary perspective. Trends Microbiol. 2008:16:2:80-88. DOI: 10.1016/j.tim.2007.12.003. PMID: 18191569.

[6] Pialoux G, Gaüzère BA, Jauréguiberry S, Strobel M: Chikungunya, an epidemic arbovirosis. Lancet Infect Dis. 2007:7:5:319-3127. DOI: 10.1016/S1473-3099(07)70107-X. PMID: 17448935.

[7] Nkoghe D, Kassa RFK, Bisvigou U, Caron M, Grard G, Leroy EM: No clinical or biological difference between chikungunya and dengue fever during the 2010 Gabonese outbreak. Infectious Disease Reports. 2012:2:4:1:e5. DOI: 10.4081/idr.2012.e5. PMID: 24470935

[8] Arya SC, Nirmala A: Apropos chikungunya virus diagnosis in the developing world: a pressing need. Expert Review of Anti-infective Therapy. 2012:10:2:121-122. DOI: 10.1586/eri.11.172. PMID:22339186

[9] Yactayo S, Staples JE, Millot V, Cibrelus L, Pardo PR: Epidemiology of chikungunya in the Americas. J Infect Dis. 2016:214:Suppl5:S441-445. DOI: 10.1093/infdis/jiw390. PMID: 27920170.

[10] Wibowo: Chikungunya history in Indonesia, A Re Emerging Illness?. Media Penelitian dan Pengembangan Kesehatan 2010:XX(Supp):S55-58. http://ejournal.litbang.kemkes.go.id/index.php/MPK/article/viewFile/748/939.

[11] Christie J: On epidemics of dengue fever: their diffusion and etiology. Ind Med Gaz. 1882:17:1: 27-28. https://www.ncbi.nlm.nih.gov/pmc/articles/PMC5900139/. PMID: 30433451.

[12] Halstead SB: Reappearance of chikungunya, formerly called dengue, in the Americas. Emerg Infect Dis. 2015:21:4:557-561. DOI: 10.3201/eid2104.141723. PMID: 25816211.

[13] Weaver SC, Forrester NL: Chikungunya: evolutionary history and recent epidemic spread. Antivir Res. 2015:120:32-39. DOI: 10.1016/j.antiviral.2015.04.016. PMID: 25979669.

[14] Porter KR, Tan R, Istary Y, Suharyono W, Sutaryo WS, Ma'Roef C, Listiyaningsih E, Kosasih H, Hueston L, et al: A serological study of chikungunya virus transmission in Yogyakarta, Indonesia: evidence for the first outbreak since 1982. Southeast Asian J Trop Med Public Health. 2004: 35(2):408-415. https://pubmed.ncbi.nlm.nih.gov/15691147/. PMID: 15691147.

[15] Ministry of Health (MoH) Indonesia. Indonesia health profile, 2005 (in Bahasa Indonesia). Directorate general disease prevention and control. MoH Indonesia: 2007.

[16] Laras K, Sukri NC, Larasati RP, Bangs MJ, Kosim R, Djauzi WT,

Master J,m Kosasih H, Hartati S, et al. Tracking the re-emergence of epidemic chikungunya virus in Indonesia. Trans R Soc Trop Med Hyg. 2005;99(2): 128-141. DOI: 10.1016/j.trstmh.2004.03.013. PMID: 15693148

[17] Ministry of Health (MoH) Indonesia. Indonesia health profile, 2014 (in Bahasa Indonesia). Directorate general disease prevention and control. MoH Indonesia: 2015.

[18] Ministry of Health (MoH) Indonesia. Indonesia health profile, 2015 (in Bahasa Indonesia). Directorate general disease prevention and control. MoH Indonesia: 2016.

[19] Ministry of Health (MoH) Indonesia. Indonesia health profile, 2013 (in Bahasa Indonesia). Directorate general disease prevention and control. MoH Indonesia: 2014.

[20] Ministry of Health (MoH) Indonesia. Indonesia health profile, 2012 (in Bahasa Indonesia). Directorate general disease prevention and control. MoH Indonesia: 2013.

[21] Ministry of Health (MoH) Indonesia. Indonesia health profile, 2011 (in Bahasa Indonesia). Directorate general disease prevention and control. MoH Indonesia: 2012.

[22] Ministry of Health (MoH) Indonesia. Indonesia health profile, 2010 (in Bahasa Indonesia). Directorate general disease prevention and control. MoH Indonesia: 2011.

[23] Ministry of Health (MoH) Indonesia. Indonesia health profile, 2009 (in Bahasa Indonesia). Directorate general disease prevention and control. MoH Indonesia: 2010.

[24] Ministry of Health (MoH) Indonesia. Indonesia health profile, 2008 (in Bahasa Indonesia). Directorate general disease prevention and control. MoH Indonesia: 2009.

[25] Ministry of Health (MoH) Indonesia. Indonesia health profile, 2007 (in Bahasa Indonesia). Directorate general disease prevention and control. MoH Indonesia: 2008.

[26] Ministry of Health (MoH) Indonesia. Indonesia health profile, 2006 (in Bahasa Indonesia). Directorate general disease prevention and control. MoH Indonesia: 2007.

[27] Mulyatno KC, Susilowati H, Yamanaka A, Soegijanto S, Konishi E: Primary isolation and phylogenetic studies of Chikungunya virus from Surabaya, Indonesia. Jpn J Infect Dis. 2012:65:1:92-94. https://pubmed.ncbi.nlm.nih.gov/22274167/. PMID: 22274167.

[28] Sasmono RT, Perkasa A, Yohan B, Haryanto S, Yudhaputri FA, Hayati RF, et al. Chikungunya detection during dengue outbreak in Sumatra, Indonesia: Clinical Manifestations and Virological Profile. Am J Trop Med Hyg. 2017; 97:5:1393-1398. DOI: 10.4269/ajtmh.16-0935. PMID: 29016291.

[29] Weaver SC, Reisen WK: Present and future arboviral threats. Antivir Res. 2010:85:2:328-3245. Doi: 10.1016/j.antiviral.2009.10.008. PMID: 19857523.

[30] Shragai T, Tesla B, Murdock C, Harrington LC: Zika and chikungunya: mosquito-borne viruses in a changing world. Ann N Y Acad Sci. 2017: 1399:1:61-77. DOI: 10.1111/nyas.13306. PMID: 28187236

[31] Robinson MC: An epidemic of virus disease in Southern Province, Tanganyika territory, in 1952-53. I. Clinical features. Trans R Soc Trop Med Hyg. 1955:49:1:28-32. DOI: 10.1016/0035-9203(55)90080-8. PMID: 14373834.

[32] Lumsden WH: An epidemic of virus disease in Southern Province, Tanganyika territory, in 1952-53. II.

General description and epidemiology. Trans R Soc Trop Med Hyg. 1955:49:1:33-57. DOI: 10.1016/0035-9203(55)90081-x. PMID: 14373835

[33] Weaver SC, Lecuit M: Chikungunya virus and the global spread of a mosquito-borne disease. N. Engl J Med. 2015:372:13:1231-1239. DOI: 10.1056/NEJMra1406035. PMID: 25806915

[34] WHO: Outbreak and spread of chikungunya. Wkly Epidemiol Rec. 2007; 82:47:409-415. https://pubmed.ncbi.nlm.nih.gov/18035647/. PMID: 18035647

[35] Renault P, Solet JL, Sissoko D, Balleydier E, Larrieu S, Filleul L, Lassalle C, Thiria J, Rachou E, de Valk H, et al: A major epidemic of chikungunya virus infection on Reunion Island, France, 2005-2006. Am J Trop Med Hyg. 2007:77:4:727-731. https://pubmed.ncbi.nlm.nih.gov/17978079/. PMID: 17978079.

[36] Jain M, Rai S, Chakravarti A: Chikungunya: a review. Trop Dr. 2008:38:2:70-72. DOI: 10.1258/td.2007.070019. PMID: 18453487

[37] Beesoon S, Funkhouser E, Kotea N, Spielman A, Robich RM: Chikungunya fever, Mauritius, 2006. Emerg Infect Dis. 2008:14:2:337-338. DOI: 10.3201/eid1402.071024. PMID: 18258136

[38] Maha MS, Susilarini NK, Hariastuti NI: Chikungunya virus mutation, Indonesia, 2011. Emerg Infect Dis. 2015:212:379-381. DOI: 10.3201/eid2102.141121. PMID: 25625600.

[39] Razmy A: Clinical features of chikungunya infection in Sri Lanka. Asian Pac J Trop Dis. 2014:42:131-134. DOI: 10.1016/S2222-1808(14)60329-7. PMCID: PMC4032055

[40] Rianthavorn P, Prianantathavorn K, Wuttirattanakowit N, Theamboonlers A, Poovorawan Y: An outbreak of chikungunya in southern Thailand from 2008 to 2009 caused by African strains with A226V mutation. Int J Infect Dis. 2010:14:E161–E165. DOI: 10.1016/j.ijid.2010.01.001. PMID: 20417142

[41] Theamboonlers A, Rianthavorn P, Praianantathavorn K, Wuttirattanakowit N, Poovorawan Y: Clinical and molecular characterization of chikungunya virus in South Thailand. Jpn J Infect Dis. 2009;62:4:303-305. https://pubmed.ncbi.nlm.nih.gov/19628911/. PMID: 19628911

[42] Sasayama M, Benjathummarak S, Kawashita N, Rukmanee P, Sangmukdanun S, Masrinoul P, Pitaksajjakul P, Puiprom O, Wuthisen P, Kurosu T, et al: Chikungunya virus was isolated in Thailand, 2010. Virus Genes. 2014;49(3):485-489. DOI: 10.1007/s11262-014-1105-5. PMID: 25113745

[43] Leo YS, Chow ALP, Tan LK, Lye DC, Lin L, Ng LC: Chikungunya outbreak, Singapore, 2008. Emerg Infect Dis. 2009;15:5:836-837. DOI: 10.3201/eid1505.081390. PMID: 19402989

[44] Gerardin P, Guernier V, Perrau J, Fianu A, Le Roux K, Grivard P, Michault A, de Lamballerie X, Flahault A, Favier F: Estimating chikungunya prevalence in La Reunion Island outbreak by serosurveys: two methods for two critical times of the epidemic. BMC Infect Dis. 2008:8:99. doi: 10.1186/1471-2334-8-99. PMID: 18662384.

[45] Dash PK, Parida MM, Santhosh SR, Verma SK, Tripathi NK, Ambuj S, Saxena P, Gupta N, Chaudhary M, Babu JP, et al: East Central South African genotype as the causative agent in reemergence of chikungunya outbreak in India. Vector-Borne Zoonot. 2007;74:519-527. DOI: 10.1089/vbz.2007.7272. PMID: 18171110

[46] Carey DE: Chikungunya and dengue: a case of mistaken identity? J Hist Med Allied Sci. 1971:26:3:243-262. DOI: 10.1093/jhmas/xxvi.3.243. PMID: 4938938.

[47] Yang CF, Su CL, Hsu TC, Chang SF, Lin CC, Huang JC, Shu PY: Imported chikungunya virus strains, Taiwan, 2006-2014. Emerg Infect Dis. 2016:22:11:1981-1984. DOI: 10.3201/eid2211.160404. PMID: 27767908.

[48] Endy TP, Chunsuttiwat S, Nisalak A, Libraty DH, Green S, Rothman AL, Vaughn DW, Ennis FA: Epidemiology of inapparent and symptomatic acute dengue virus infection: a prospective study of primary school children in Kamphaeng Phet, Thailand. Am J Epidemiol. 2002:156:1:40-51. DOI: 10.1093/aje/kwf005. PMID: 12076887.

[49] Carrillo FB, Gordon A, Harris E: Reply to Gérardin et al. Clin Infect Dis. 2018:68:1:172-1724. DOI: 10.1093/cid/ciy535. PMID: 29982451.

[50] P Ramon-Pardo, L Cibrelus, S Yactayo: Chikungunya: case definitions for acute, atypical and chronic cases. Conclusions of an expert consultation, Managua, Nicaragua, 20-21 May 2015. Wkly Epidemiol Rec. 2015:90:33:410-414. https://pubmed.ncbi.nlm.nih.gov/26281046/. PMID: 26281046.

[51] Yoon IK, Alera MT, Lago CB, Tac-An IA, Villa D, Fernandez S, Thaisomboonsuk B, Klungthong C, Levy JW, Velasco JM, et al: High rate of subclinical chikungunya virus infection and association of neutralizing antibody with protection in a prospective cohort in the Philippines. PLoS Negl Trop Dis. 2015:9:5:e0003764. DOI: 10.1371/journal.pntd.0003764. PMID: 25951202.

[52] Weaver SC, Lecuit M: Chikungunya virus and the global spread of a mosquito-borne disease. N Engl J Med. 2015:372:13:1231-1239. DOI: 10.1056/NEJMra1406035. PMID: 25806915.

[53] Mourya DT, Mishra AC: Chikungunya fever. Lancet. 2006:368:9531:186-187. DOI: 10.1016/S0140-6736(06)69017-X. PMID: 16844472

[54] Gerardin P, Couderc T, Bintner M, Tournebize P, Renouil M, Lemant J, Boisson V, Borgherini G, Staikowsky F, Schramm F, et al: Chikungunya virusassociated encephalitis: a cohort study on La Reunion Island, 2005-2009. Neurology. 2016:86:1:94-102. DOI: 10.1212/WNL.0000000000002234. PMID: 26609145.

[55] Mehta R, Gerardin P, de Brito CAA, Soares CN, Ferreira MLB, Solomon T: The neurological complications of chikungunya virus: a systematic review. Rev Med Virol. 2018:28:3:e1978. DOI: 10.1002/rmv.1978. PMID: 29671914.

[56] Lemant J, Boisson V, Winer A, Thibault L, Andre H, Tixier F, Lemercier M, Antok E, Cresta MP, Grivard P, et al: Serious acute chikungunya virus infection requiring intensive care during the Reunion Island outbreak in 2005-2006. Crit Care Med. 2008:36:9:2536-2541. DOI: 10.1097/CCM.0b013e318183f2d2. PMID: 18679124.

[57] Rajapakse S, Rodrigo C, Rajapakse A: Atypical manifestations of chikungunya infection. Trans R Soc Trop Med Hyg. 2010:104:2:89-96. DOI: 10.1016/j.trstmh.2009.07.031. PMID: 19716149

[58] Cerny T, Schwarz M, Schwarz U, Lemant J, Gerardin P, Keller E: The range of neurological complications in chikungunya fever. Neurocrit Care. 2017:27:3: 447-457. DOI: 10.1007/s12028-017-0413-8. PMID: 28741102.

[59] Chua HH, Abdul Rashid K, Law WC, Hamizah A, Chem YK,

Khairul AH, Chua KB: A fatal case of chikungunya virus infection with liver involvement. Med J Malaysia. 2010:65:1:83-84. https://pubmed.ncbi.nlm.nih.gov/21265260/. PMID: 21265260

[60] Mercado M, Acosta-Reyes J, Parra E, Guzman L, Beltran M, Gasque P, MejiaGarcia C, Viasus D: Renal involvement in fatal cases of chikungunya virus infection. J Clin Virol. 2018:103:16-18. DOI: 10.1016/j.jcv.2018.03.009. PMID: 29604514.

[61] Rolle A, Schepers K, Cassadou S, Curlier E, Madeux B, Hermann-Storck C, Fabre I, Lamaury I, Tressieres B, Thiery G, et al: Severe sepsis and septic shock associated with chikungunya virus infection, Guadeloupe, 2014. Emerg Infect Dis. 2016:22:5:891-894. doi: 10.3201/eid2205.151449. PMID: 27088710.

[62] Gauri LA, Ranwa BL, Nagar K, Vyas A, Fatima Q: Post chikungunya brain stem encephalitis. J Assoc Physicians India. 2012:60:68-70. https://pubmed.ncbi.nlm.nih.gov/23029750/. PMID: 23029750.

[63] Hoz JM, Bayona B, Viloria S, Accini JL, Juan-Vergara HS, Viasus D: Fatal cases of chikungunya virus infection in Colombia: diagnostic and treatment challenges. J Clin Virol. 2015:69:27-29. DOI: 10.1016/j.jcv.2015.05.021. PMID: 26209372.

[64] Gerardin P, Samperiz S, Ramful D, Boumahni B, Bintner M, Alessandri JL, Carbonnier M, Tiran-Rajaoefera I, Beullier G, Boya I, et al: Neurocognitive outcome of children exposed to perinatal mother-to-child chikungunya virus infection: the CHIMERE cohort study on Reunion Island. PLoS Negl Trop Dis. 2014:8:7:e2996. DOI: 10.1371/journal.pntd.0002996. PMID: 25033077.

[65] Van Aalst M, Nelen CM, Goorhuis A, Stijnis C, Grobusch MP: Long-term sequelae of chikungunya virus disease: a systematic review. Travel Med Infect Dis. 2017:15:8-22. DOI: 10.1016/j.tmaid.2017.01.004. PMID: 28163198

[66] Zaid A, Gerardin P, Taylor A, Mostafavi H, Malvy D, Mahalingam S: Chikungunya arthritis: implications of acute and chronic inflammation mechanisms on disease management. Arthritis Rheumatol. 2018:70:4:484-495. DOI: 10.1002/art.40403. PMID: 29287308.

[67] Paixao ES, Rodrigues LC, Costa M, Itaparica M, Barreto F, Gerardin P, Teixeira MG: Chikungunya chronic disease: a systematic review and meta-analysis. Trans R Soc Trop Med Hyg. 2018:112:7:301-316. DOI: 10.1093/trstmh/try063. PMID: 30007303.

[68] Rodriguez-Morales AJ, Cardona-Ospina JA, Fernanda Urbano-Garzon S, Sebastian Hurtado-Zapata J: Prevalence of post-chikungunya infection chronic inflammatory arthritis: a systematic review and meta-analysis. Arthritis Care Res (Hoboken). 2016:68:12:1849-1858. DOI: 10.1002/acr.22900. PMID: 27015439

[69] Ministry of Health (MoH) Indonesia. Indonesia health profile, 2019 (in Bahasa Indonesia). Directorate general disease prevention and control. MoH Indonesia: 2020.

[70] Knope KE, Doggett SL, Kurucz N, Johansen CA, Nicholson J, Feldman R, Sly A, Hobby M, El Saadi D, Muller M, et al: Arboviral diseases and malaria in Australia, 2011-12: annual report of the National Arbovirus and malaria advisory committee. Commun Dis Intell Q Rep. 2014:38:2:E122–E142. https://pubmed.ncbi.nlm.nih.gov/25222207/. PMID: 25222207.

[71] Knope KE, Kurucz N, Doggett SL, Muller M, Johansen CA, Feldman R,

Hobby M, Bennett S, Sly A, Lynch S, et al: Arboviral diseases and malaria in Australia, 2012-13: annual report of the National Arbovirus and malaria advisory committee. Commun Dis Intell Q Rep. 2016:401:E17–E47. https://pubmed.ncbi.nlm.nih.gov/27080023/. PMID: 27080023

[72] Knope KE, Muller M, Kurucz N, Doggett SL, Feldman R, Johansen CA, Hobby M, Bennett S, Lynch S, Sly A, et al: Arboviral diseases and malaria in Australia, 2013-14: annual report of the National Arbovirus and malaria advisory committee. Commun Dis Intell Q Rep. 2016;40:3:E400–E436. https://pubmed.ncbi.nlm.nih.gov/28278416/. PMID: 28278416

[73] Knope KE, Muller M, Kurucz N, Doggett SL, Feldman R, Johansen CA, Hobby M, Bennett S, Lynch S, Sly A, et al: Arboviral diseases and malaria in Australia, 2014-15: annual report of the National Arbovirus and malaria advisory committee. Commun Dis Intell Q Rep. 2019:15:43. DOI: 10.33321/cdi.2019.43.14. PMID: 30982295.

[74] Harnett GB, Bucens MR: Isolation of chikungunya virus in Australia. Med J Aust. 1990:152:6:328-329. https://pubmed.ncbi.nlm.nih.gov/2156139/. PMID: 2156139.

[75] Wright P, Fitzsimmons GJ, Johansen CA, Whelan PI, Co NAMA: Arboviral diseases and malaria in Australia, 2009-10: annual report of the National Arbovirus and malaria advisory committee. Commun Dis Intell Q Rep. 2012:36:1:70-81. https://pubmed.ncbi.nlm.nih.gov/23153083/. PMID: 23153083

[76] Knope K, Whelan P, Smith D, Johansen C, Moran R, Doggett S, Sly A, Hobby M, Kurucz N, Wright P, et al: Arboviral diseases and malaria in Australia, 2010-11: annual report of the National Arbovirus and malaria advisory committee. Commun Dis Intell Q Rep. 2013:37:1:E1–E20. https://pubmed.ncbi.nlm.nih.gov/23692155/. PMID: 23692155

[77] Fitzsimmons GJ, Wright P, Johansen CA, Whelan PI, Ad NAM: Arboviral diseases and malaria in Australia, 2007/08: annual report of the National Arbovirus and malaria advisory committee. Commun Dis Intell Q Rep. 2009:33:2:155-169. https://pubmed.ncbi.nlm.nih.gov/19877534/. PMID: 19877534.

[78] Shu PY, Yang CF, Su CL, Chen CY, Chang SF, Tsai KH, Cheng CH, Huang JH. Two imported chikungunya cases, Taiwan. Emerg Infect Dis. 2008:14:8:1326-1327. DOI: 10.320l/eid1408.071304. PMID: 18680674.

[79] Huang JH, Yang CF, Su CL, Chang SF, Cheng CH, Yu SK, Lin CC, Shu PY: Imported chikungunya virus strains, Taiwan, 2006-2009. Emerg Infect Dis. 2009:15:11:1854-1856. DOI: 10.3201/eid1511.090398. PMID: 19891886.

[80] Kobashi K, Kobayashi T, Nakamura-Uchiyama F, Ohnishi K: A Japanese patient with chikungunya fever returning from Flores Island, Indonesia. Kansenshogaku Zasshi. 2010:84:4:457-459. DOI: 10.11150/kansenshogakuzasshi.84.457. PMID: 20715557.

[81] Mizuno Y, Kato Y, Takeshita N, Ujiie M, Kobayashi T, Kanagawa S, Kudo K, Lim CK, Takasaki T: Clinical and radiological features of imported chikungunya fever in Japan: a study of six cases at the National Center for Global Health and medicine. J Infect Chemother. 2011:17:3:419-423. DOI: 10.1007/s10156-010-0124-y. PMID: 20862507.

[82] Volk SM, Chen R, Tsetsarkin KA, Adams AP, Garcia TI, Sall AA, Nasar F, Schuh AJ, Holmes EC, Higgs S, et al: Genome-scale phylogenetic analyses of

chikungunya virus reveal independent emergences of recent epidemics and Various evolutionary rates. J Virol. 2010:84:13:6497-6504. DOI: 10.1128/JVI.01603-09. PMID: 20410280.

[83] Shchelkanov M, L'Vov DK, Kolobukhina LV, Al'khovskii SV, Shchetinin AM, Saifullin MA, Kruzhkova IS, Aristova VA, Morozova TV, Samokhvalov EI, et al: Isolation of the chikungunya virus in Moscow from the Indonesian visitor (September, 2013). Vopr Virusol. 2014:59:3:28-34. https://pubmed.ncbi.nlm.nih.gov/25335416/. PMID: 25335416

[84] Panning M, Grywna K, van Esbroeck M, Emmerich P, Drosten C: Chikungunya fever in travelers returning to Europe from the Indian Ocean region, 2006. Emerg Infect Dis. 2008:14:3:416-422. DOI: 10.3201/eid1403.070906. PMID: 18325256.

[85] Chaves T, Pellini A, Mascheretti M, Jahnel M, Ribeiro A, Rodrigues S, Vasconcelos P, Boulos M: Travelers as sentinels for chikungunya fever, Brazil. Emerg Infect Dis. 2012:18:3:529-530. DOI: 10.3201/eid1803.110838. PMID: 22377013.

[86] Roth A, Hoy D, Horwood PF, Ropa B, Hancock T, Guillaumot L, Rickart K, Frison P, Pavlin B, Souares Y: Preparedness for threat of chikungunya in the pacific. Emerg Infect Dis. 2014:20:8:e130696. DOI: 10.3201/eid2008.130696. PMID: 25062306.

[87] Scholte FE, Tas A, Martina BE, Cordioli P, Narayanan K, Makino S, Snijder EJ, van Hemert MJ. Characterization of synthetic chikungunya viruses based on the consensus sequence of recent E1-226V isolates. PLoS One. 2013:8:8:e71047. DOI: 10.1371/journal.pone.0071047. PMID: 23936484.

[88] Wolfel S, Vollmar P, Poluda D, Zange S, Antwerpen MH, Loscher T, Dobler G: Complete genome sequence of a chikungunya virus imported from Bali to Germany. Genome announcements. 2015:3:2: e00164-e00115. DOI: 10.1128/genomeA.00164-15. PMID: 25814598.

[89] Environmental Systems Research Institute (ESRI). ArcGIS Release 10.1. [Internet]. Available from: https://www.esri.com/news/arcnews/spring12articles/introducing-arcgis-101.html.

[90] Kearse M, Moir R, Wilson A, Stones-Havas S, Cheung M, Sturrock S, Buxton S, Cooper A, Markowitz S, Duran C, et al: Geneious basic: An integrated and extendable desktop software platform for the organization and analysis of sequence data. Bioinformatics. 2012;28(12): 1647-1649. DOI: 10.1093/bioinformatics/bts199. PMID: 22543367.

[91] Sari K, Myint K, Andayani A, Adi P, Dhenni R, Perkasa D, Maroef C, Witaria N, Megawati D, Powers A, et al: Chikungunya fever outbreak identified in North Bali, Indonesia. Trans R Soc Trop Med Hyg. 2017:111:7:325-327. DOI: 10.1093/trstmh/trx054. PMID: 29029262

[92] Ng LC, Tan LK, Tan CH, Tan SS, Hapuarachchi HC, Pok KY, Lai YL, Lam-Phua SG, Bucht G, Lin RT, et al: Entomologic and virologic investigation of chikungunya, Singapore. Emerg Infect Dis. 2009:15:8:1243-1249. DOI: 10.3201/eid1508.081486. PMID: 19751586.

[93] Harapan Harapan, Alice Michie, Mudatsir Mudatsir, Roy Nusa, Benediktus Yohan, Abram Luther Wagner, R. Tedjo Sasmono, Allison Imrie: Chikungunya virus infection in Indonesia: a systematic review and evolutionary analysis BMC Infect Dis. 2019:19:243:1-20 https://www.ncbi.nlm.nih.gov/pmc/articles/PMC6417237/. PMID: 30866835

[94] Riswari SF, Ma'roef CN, Djauhari H, Kosasih H, Perkasa A, Yudhaputri FA, Artika IM, Williams M, Van der Ven A, Myint KS, et al: Study of viremic profile in febrile specimens of chikungunya in Bandung, Indonesia. J Clin Virol. 2016:74:61-65. DOI: 10.1016/j.jcv.2015.11.017. PMID: 26679829.

[95] Shchelkanov M, L'Vov DK, Kolobukhina LV, Al'khovskii SV, Shchetinin AM, Saifullin MA, Kruzhkova IS, Aristova VA, Morozova TV, Samokhvalov EI, et al: Isolation of the chikungunya virus in Moscow from the Indonesian visitor (September, 2013). Vopr Virusol. 2014:59:3:28-34. https://pubmed.ncbi.nlm.nih.gov/25335416/. PMID: 25335416

[96] Sasmono R, Perkasa A, Yohan B, Haryanto S, Yudhaputri FA, Hayati R, Maaroef C, Ledermann J, Myint K, Powers A. Chikungunya deterection during dengue outbreak in Sumatera, Indonesia: clinical manifestatation and virological profile. Am J Trop Med Hyg. 2017:97:5:1393-1398. DOI: 10.4269/ajtmh.16-0935. PMID: 29016291

[97] Kosasih H, de Mast Q, Widjaja S, Sudjana P, Antonjaya U, Ma'roef C, Riswari SF, Porter KR, Burgess TH, Alisjahbana B, et al: Evidence for endemic chikungunya virus infections in Bandung, Indonesia. PLoS Negl Trop Dis. 2013:7:10:e2483. DOI: 10.1371/journal.pntd.0002483. PMID: 24205417.

[98] Grandadam M, Caro V, Plumet S, Thiberge JM, Souares Y, Failloux AB, Tolou HJ, Budelot M, Cosserat D, Leparc-Goffart I, et al: Chikungunya virus, southeastern France. Emerg Infect Dis. 2011:17:5::910-913. DOI: 10.3201/eid1705.101873. PMID: 21529410.

[99] Powers AM, Brault AC, Tesh RB, Weaver SC: Re-emergence of chikungunya and O'nyong-nyong viruses: evidence for distinct geographical lineages and distant evolutionary relationships. J Gen Virol. 2000;81(Pt 2):471-479. DOI: 10.1099/0022-1317-81-2-471. PMID: 10644846.

[100] Harbach, Ralph. Mosquito Taxonomic Inventory [Internet]. 2015. Available from: http://mosquito-taxonomic-inventory.info/simpletaxonomy/term/8589Aedes, 18 Agustus 2015, [Accessed: 2020-12-14].

[101] Satoto TBT, Alvira Nur, Wibawa T, Diptyanusa Ajib: Controlling factors that potentially against transmission of dengue hemorrhagic fever at state elementary schools in Yogyakarta. National: Public Health Journal. 2017; 11:4: 178-184. DOI: 10.21109/kesmas.v11i4. 1248.

[102] Rueda, L. Pictorial keys for the identification of mosquitoes (diptera: culicidae) associated with dengue virus transmission. Zootaxa: Magnolia Press. 2004:589:1:60. DOI: 10.11646/zootaxa.589.1.1.

[103] Andrew J, Bar Ananya: Morphology and Morphometry of Aedes aegypti Adult Mosquito. Annual Research and Review in Biology. 2013:1:1: 52-69. https://www.journalarrb.com/index.php/ARRB/article/view/24618.

[104] Satoto TBT, Pascawati NA, Wibawa T, Frutos Roger, Maguin Sylvie, Mulyawan I Kadek, Wardana Ali: Entomological index and home environment contribution to dengue hemorrhagic fever in Mataram City, Indonesia. 2020: 15:1: 32-39. DOI: http://dx.doi.org/10.21109/kesmas.v15i1.3294.

[105] Gratz NG: Critical review of the vector status of *Aedes albopictus*. Medical and veterinary entomology. 2013: 18: 3: 215-227. DOI: https://doi.org/10.1111/j.0269-283X.2004.00513.x. PMID: 15347388.

[106] Hawley WA: The biology of Aedes albopictus. Journal of the American Mosquito Control Association Supplement. 1988:1:1-39. https://pubmed.ncbi.nlm.nih.gov/3068349/. PMID: 3068349.

[107] Bova JE. Morphological differentiation of eggs and comparative efficacy of oviposition and gravid traps for Aedes vectors at different habitats [thesis]. Virginia: Masters of Science in Entomology Blacksburg; 2014.

[108] Schlaeger DA, Fuchs, MS: Effect of DOPA-decarboxylase inhibition of Aedes aegypti eggs: evidence fo sclerotization. Journal of Insect Physiology. 1974:20:2:349-357. DOI: 10.1016/0022-1910(74)90066-3. PMID: 4815641

[109] Briscoe MS: *Aedes aegypti* (L) the yellow fever mosquito: Its life history, bionomics and structure. Journal of the National Medical Association. 1962: 54:1: 132. PMCID: PMC2642088.

[110] DS Kettle. Medical and Veterinary Entomology. Croom Helm Ltd. Beckenham: UK; 1984. 658p. ISBN: 0856648396.

[111] Rodhain F, Rosen. Mosquito vectors and dengue virus-vector relationships. In: D.J Gubler. And G. Kuno (eds) Dengue and Dengue Hemorrhagic fever. CAB International: New York; 1997. 61-88p.

[112] Goma LKH. The mosquito. Hutchinson and Co. Ltd: London; 1966. 144p. Record Number: 19661000683.

[113] RF Harwood, MT James. Entomology in human and animal health. 7th ed. Bailliere Tindall: New York USA; 1979. ISBN : 0023516003.

[114] Service MW. Medical entomology for students. 3rd ed. Liverpool School of Tropical Medicine. Liverpool: UK; 1996. ISBN: 052154775.

[115] HO, BC, KL Chan, YC Chan. III. Control of Aedes vectors. di The biology and bionomic of *Aedes albopictus* (Skuse). Proceedings 1st SEAMEO Workshop. Singapore; 1972.

[116] SNR Saleeza, Y Norma-Rashid, M Sofian-Azirun: Mosquitoes larval breeding habitat in urban and suburban areas, Peninsular Malaysia. World Academy of Science, Engineering and Technology. 2011:5:10:569-573.

[117] JJ Wilson, SP Sevarkodiyone: Spatial and temporal distribution of mosquitoes (Culicidae) in Virudhunagar district, Tamil Nadu, South India. International Journal of Mosquito Research. 2014:1:3:4-9. ISSN: 2348-5906.

[118] Satoto TBT, Dwiputro AH, Risdwiyanto RN, Hakim AUF, Pascawati NA, Diptyanusa A: Prediction model of dengue hemorrhagic fever transmission to enhance early warning system in Gergunung Village, Klaten District, Central Java: Journal of Medical Science. 2019:51:3:258-269. DOI: 10.19106/JMedSci005103201909.

[119] A Philbert, JN Ijumba: Preferred breeding habitats of *Aedes aegypti* (Diptera-Culicidae) mosquito and its public health implications in Dares Salaam, Tanzani. Journal of Environmental Research and Management. 2013:4:10:344-351. ISSN: 2141-7466

[120] Edman JD, Strickman D, Kittayapong P, Scott TW: Female *Aedes aegypti* (Diptera: Culicidae) in Thailand rarely feed on sugar. Journal of Medical Entomology. 1992:29:6:1035-1038. DOI: 10.1093/jmedent/29.6.1035. PMID: 1460619

[121] Paupy C, Delatte H, Bagny L, Corbel V, Fontenille D: *Aedes albopictus*, an arbovirus vector: from the darkness to the light. Microbes Infect. 2009: 11:14-15:1177-1785. DOI: 10.1016/j.micinf.2009.05.005 PMID: .

[122] Delatte H, Gimonneau G, Triboire A, Fontenille D: Influence of temperature on immature development, survival, longevity, fecundity, and gonotrophic cycles of *Aedes albopictus*, vector of chikungunya and dengue in the Indian Ocean. J Med Entomol. 2009:46:1:33-41. DOI: 10.1603/033.046.0105. PMID: 19198515.

[123] WHO. Dengue and severe dengue [Internet]. 2019. Available from: https://www.who.int/news-room/q-a-detail/dengue-and-severe-dengue [Accessed: 2020-12-14].

[124] Nelson MJ. *Aedes aegypti*: Biology and Ecology. [Internet]. 1986. Available from: https://iris.paho.org/handle/10665.2/28514?show=full [Accessed: 2020-12-14].

[125] WHO. Mosquitos and other biting Diptera. Jan A. Rozendaal editors. Vector Control - Methods for Use by Individuals and Communities. 1st ed. World Health Organization; 1997. p. 7-28. https://apps.who.int/iris/handle/10665/41968.

[126] Pascawati NA, Pohan N. Description of the density and potential places ofthe breeding of aedes sp. Larvae in public areas in the working area of the Public Health Center of Umbulharjo, Yogyakarta City. Jurnal Formil (Forum Ilmiah) KesMas Respati: 1(2); 109-120. ISSN 2502-5570.

[127] Chan, Y. C, B. C. Ho, and K. L. Chan. 1971. Aedes aegypti (L.) and Aedes albopictus (Skuse) in Singapore City. 5. Observations in relation to dengue haemorrhagic fever. Bull World Health Organ. 1971:44:5:651-657. https://pubmed.ncbi.nlm.nih.gov/5316749/. PMID: 5316749.

[128] Djoni Djunaedi. Demam Berdarah. 1st ed. UMM Press: Malang: 2006. 26 p.

[129] DW Jenkins, CC Hassett: Dispersal and Flight Range of subarctic Mosquitoes marked with Radiophosphorus. Can J Zool. 1951: 29:3:178-187. DOI: 10.1139/z51-017.

[130] N Becker, D Petric, M Zgomba, C Boase, M Madon, C Dahl, A Kaiser. Mosquitoes and Their Control. 2nd ed. Springer Heidelberg: Dordrecht: New York; 2010. 577 p. DOI: 10.1007/978-3-540-92874-4.

[131] C Kaufmann, H Briegel: Flight performance of the malaria vectors *Anopheles gambiae* and Anopheles atroparvus J Vector Ecol. 2004:29:1:140-153. https://pubmed.ncbi.nlm.nih.gov/15266751/PMID: 15266751.

[132] Bringhton SW, Prozesky OW, Harpe AL de la: Chikungunya virus infection. A retrospective study of 107 cases. S Afr Med J. 1983:63:9:313-315. https://pubmed.ncbi.nlm.nih.gov/6298956/. PMID: 6298956

[133] Soegeng Soegijanto. Collection of Papers on Tropical Diseases and Infections in Indonesia (In Bahasa Indonesia). 1st ed. Airlangga University Press: Surabaya; 2004. 63 p.

[134] Chhabra M, Mittal V, Bhattacharya D, Rana Uvs, Lal S: Chikungunya fever: a re-emerging viral infection. Indian J Med Microbial. 2008: 26:1:5-12. DOI: 10.4103/0255-0857.38850. PMID: 18227590.

[135] WHO. Chikungunya [Internet]. Available from:https://www.who.int/news-room/fact-sheets/detail/chikungunya [Accessed: 2020-12-20].

[136] WHO. Preparedness and response for Chikungunya Virus Introduction in the Americas. Center for Disease Control and Prevention: Pan American Health Organization: Washington: 2011. ISBN: 978-92-75-11632-6.

[137] Brighton SW: Chloroquine phosphate treatment of chronic chikungunya arthritis. An open pilot

study. S Afr Med J. 1984:66:6:217-218. https://pubmed.ncbi.nlm.nih.gov/6087474/. PMID: 6087474

[138] De Lamballerie X, Boisson V, Reynier JC, Enault Sebastien, Charrel Remi N, Flahault, Roques Pierre, Grand Roger Le. On chikungunya acute infection and chloroquine treatment. Vector Borne Zoonotic Dis. 2008:8:6:837-839. DOI: 10.1089/vbz.2008.0049. PMID: 18620511.

[139] Cordel H, Quatresous I, Paquet C, Couturier E: Imported cases of chikungunya in metropolitan France, April 2005 - February 2006. Euro Surveill. 2006:11:4:E060420.3. DOI: 10.2807/esw.11.16.02944-en. PMID: 16809828.

[140] US DHHS. Biosafety in microbiological and biomedical laboratories. 4th ed. Washington: DC: US Government Printing Office; 1999.

[141] Ministry of Health (MoH) Indonesia. Guidelines for the prevention and control of chikungunya fever in Indonesia (in Bahasa Indonesia). Directorate general disease prevention and control. MoH Indonesia: 2017.

[142] Gerardin P, Barau G, Michault A, Michault Alain, Bintner Marc, Randrianaivo Hanitra, Choker Ghassan, Lenglet Yann Touret Yasmina, Bouveret Anne: Multidisciplinary prospective study of mother-to-child chikungunya virus infections on the island of La Réunion. PLoS Med. 2008:5:3:e60. DOI: 10.1371/journal.pmed.0050060. PMID: 18351797.

[143] Garjito TW Ambar, Hidajat MC, Kinansi RS, Anggraeni YM, Mujiyanto, Tripsilowati W, Jastal, Ristiyanto, Satoto TBT: Stegomyia indices and risk of dengue transmission: A lack of Correlation. Front. Public Health. 2020:8:328:1-13. DOi: 10.3389/fpubh.2020.00328.

[144] Barrera R, Delgado N, Jimenez M, Villalobos I, Romero I: Stratification of a hyperendemic city in hemorrhagic dengue. Rev Panam Salud Publica. 2000:8:4:225-233. DOI: 10.1590/s1020-49892000000900001. PMID: 11141964.

[145] Mulyaningsih Budi, Umniyati SR, Satoto TBT, Diptyanusa Ajib, Selin Yahiddin: Insecticide resistance and possible mechanisms of *Aedes aegypti* (Diptera: Culicidae) in Yogyakarta, Indonesia. Journal of the Medical Science. 2018: 50:1:24-32. DOI: 10.19106/JMedSci005001201803.

[146] Sukesi TY, Supriyati S, Satoto TBT: Community Empowerment in Dengue Hemorrhagic Fever Control (Literature Review). Journal of Disease Vector. 2018:12:2:67-77. DOI: 10.22435/vektorp.v12i2.294.

[147] Sulistyawati S, Astuti FD, Umniyati SR, Satoto TBT, Lazuardi L, Nilsson M, Rocklov Joacim, Andersson C, Holmner A: Dengue vector control through community empowerment: lessons learned from a community-based study in Yogyakarta, Indonesia. 2019:16:6:1013. DOI: 10.3390/ijerph16061013. PMID: 30897770.

[148] Morrison AC, Zielinski-Gutierrez E, Scott TW, Rosenberg R: Defining challenges and proposing solutions for control of the virus vector *Aedes aegypti*. PLoS Med. 2008:5:3:e68. DOI: 10.1371/journal.pmed.0050068. PMID: 18351798.

Section 4

Transmission

Chapter 4

Chikungunya Virus Transmission

Lucille Lyaruu

Abstract

Chikungunya virus (CHIKV) is a mosquito-borne *Alphavirus* that causes Chikungunya fever (CHIKF) in humans. In 1952, the CHIKV was found in East Africa in a sylvatic and urban cycle between *Aedes* mosquitoes, and human and nonhuman primates in tropical regions. Since 2004, CHIKF has spread rapidly in Asia, Africa, Europe, and the Americas. Both *Aedes aegypti* and *Aedes albopictus* are known to be arboviral mosquito vectors of CHIKV. *Ae. aegypti* is mostly found within the tropics, whereby *Ae. albopictus* also occurs in temperate and cold temperate regions. Host-seeking female mosquitoes are infected after feeding on a viremic animal. The replication of CHIKV happens in the midgut and then enters the hemocoel before disseminating to the salivary glands of the mosquito. The disseminated virus can be transmitted by injecting infectious saliva into the host skin during blood feeding. In the naïve host body, CHIKV replicates in the dermal fibroblasts through blood circulation, and disseminates to other parts of the body such as brain cells, kidney, heart, lymphoid tissues, liver, and joints. Symptoms of CHIKV infection include high fever, rigors, headache, photophobia, and maculopapular rash. It is advised to avoid mosquito bites; also, larvae management systems should be applied in endemic environments.

Keywords: Chikungunya virus, Chikungunya fever, *Aedes aegypti*, *Aedes albopictus*, *Alphavirus*

1. Introduction

Chikungunya fever (CHIKF) is an arthropod-borne viral disease caused by the Chikungunya virus (CHIKV) which belongs to the Togaviridae family of genus *Alphavirus*. CHIKV is closely related to other Alphaviruses, including Ross River virus, Barmah Forest virus, O'nyong'nyong virus, the Sindbis group of viruses, and the Mayaro virus, all of which are known to cause arthritis. CHIKV has three genotypes that show different distribution geographically; Asian, West African, and East African [1].

The term "Chikungunya" was derived from the local word in the Makonde tribe based in the Southeastern part of Tanzania, meaning "disease that bends up the joints and causing pains" [2]. The CHIKV infection was first identified as an outbreak with an incidence rate estimated at 23%. It was reported for the period going from July 1952 to March 1953 in the Newala and Masasi districts in Southern Tanzania. The virus was isolated in early 1953 from the blood of several febrile patients. The CHIKV was initially found in East Africa in a sylvatic cycle between forest-dwelling *Aedes* mosquitoes and nonhuman primates in tropical and subtropical regions. Otherwise, a few isolations of CHIKV have been reported in other mammalian species including bats and squirrels [3].

2. Chikungunya vectors

2.1 Distribution

CHIKV is primarily transmitted by Stegomyia vector mosquitoes that belong to genus *Aedes*. *Aedes* mosquitoes are also known to be vectors of the dengue and the Zika fever viruses. Both *Ae. aegypti* and *Ae. albopictus* have been implicated in large outbreaks of CHIKF though they differ in distribution and occurrence. *Ae. aegypti* is mainly found within the tropics and subtropics regions. Furthermore, *Ae. albopictus* occurs in temperate and even cold temperate regions [4].

In Asia and the Indian Ocean regions, the main CHIKV vectors are *Ae. aegypti* and *Ae. albopictus*. In Africa, there is a larger range of *Aedes* species that are known to transmit CHIKV including *Ae. furcifer-taylori*, *Ae. vittatus*, *Ae. fulgens*, *Ae. luteocephalus*, *Ae. dalzieli*, *Ae. vigilax*, and *Ae. camptorhynchites*. In addition, *Culex annulirostris*, *Mansonia uniformis*, and *Anopheles* mosquitoes have occasionally been incriminated [5].

2.2 Ecology

The *Aedes* mosquitoes are known as container breeders meant that a female mosquito can lay eggs on collected water in an artificial and/or natural container. The *Ae. albopictus* species thrives in a wider range of natural water-filled breeding sites than *Ae. aegypti*, including coconut husks, cocoa pods, bamboo stumps, tree holes, plant axils, and rock pools, in addition to artificial containers such as vehicle tires, roof gutters, water storage buckets, and saucers beneath plant pots [6].

Ae. aegypti is more closely associated with human habitation and uses indoor breeding sites, including flower vases, water storage vessels, and concrete water tanks in bathrooms, as well as the same artificial outdoor habitats as *Ae. albopictus* [7, 8].

Adult, female mosquitoes can lay eggs on the inner walls of the containers with water, above the waterline. Eggs stick singly to container walls like glue and can survive drying out for up to 8 months, enabling them to survive cold winters and other adverse climatic conditions [9]. *Aedes* larvae hatch from the eggs and live in water, typically hanging upside down at an angle from the water surface, where they use a short thick respiratory siphon to take up oxygen from the air above the water. Larvae mature through four instars (stages), in the last stage developing into pupae, which subsequently change into adults that emerge at the water's surface. Within 2 days of emerging, adult *Aedes* mosquitoes' mate and females subsequently consume their first blood meal. *Aedes* mosquitoes prefer feeding on human blood during the daytime from early morning to a late afternoon outdoor, but *Ae. aegypti* can be active feeding indoor [10].

2.3 Host-seeking and blood-feeding behavior

Aedes mosquitoes are aggressive and silent, and prefer to feed outdoor during the daytime. *Ae. aegypti*, an important vector of human infectious diseases, shows a strong preference for human blood meals when compared to many other mosquitoes which feed on warm-blooded animals [11]. Temperature and nutrition are the environmental factors that affect mostly mosquito population growth. Biological signals can be captured from the mosquitoes surrounding environment and sensed through olfaction and other chemosensory organs, which play a major role in the modulation of mosquito behaviors such as hosts seeking, feeding, mating, oviposition, and reception of cues. Olfactory responses are initiated by activation of olfactory sensory neurons (OSNs) localized mainly on antennae, maxillary palps, mouthparts, and tarsi. These sensory appendages may perceive extremely diverse extrinsic stimuli, such as volatile and nonvolatile odors or pheromones, temperature, humidity, mild or noxious touch, gravity, to activate a complex mix of mosquito perception pathways [12].

Ae. aegypti and *Ae. albopictus* are the competent vectors of various infectious diseases, and their body size is much affected by temperature and nutrition. Mosquito body size is known to influence several attributes of vector ecology, fecundity, and multiple blood feeding [13]. Multiple feeding increases the risk of transmission by increasing the frequency of host contacts and can be of two types including supplementary and interrupted feeding. Supplementary feeding can happen as nutritional reserve depletion in teneral females, whereby interrupted feeding happens as host defense [14].

3. Chikungunya virus

3.1 Distribution

Since 2004, Chikungunya has spread rapidly and been identified in over 60 countries throughout Asia, Africa, Europe, and the Americas. In 2007, local transmission was reported for the first time in Europe and more specifically in north-eastern Italy where a localized outbreak of 197 cases were recorded. In 2014, Europe faced its highest Chikungunya burden, with almost 1500 cases of which France and the UK were the most affected. France also confirmed four cases of locally-acquired Chikungunya infection in the southern part of the country [15].

In the year 2013, the first documented outbreak of Chikungunya with the autochthonous transmission in the Americas occurred [16]. In 2016, there were a total of 349,936 suspected cases and 146,914 laboratory-confirmed cases reported to the Pan African Health Organization (PAHO) regional office, which represented half of the burden compared to the previous year. In 2017, European Centre for Diseases Prevention and Control (ECDC) reported a total of 10 countries, with 548 cases of Chikungunya, of which 84% were confirmed cases. Italy bore more than 50% of the Chikungunya burden.

In Africa and Asia, Chikungunya outbreaks were also reported in Senegal (2015), Kenya (2004 and 2016), Tanzania (2008), Sudan (2018), Yemen (2019), and more recently in Cambodia and Chad (2020) [15–17].

3.2 Transmission

CHIKV can be transmitted in a sylvatic, enzootic, and urban cycle involving humans, nonhumans, and *Ae. aegypti* and *Ae. albopictus* mosquito species as shown in **Figure 1**.

In Africa, circulation in sylvatic, enzootic cycles involves several species of arboreal mosquito vectors that transmit among diverse nonhuman primates and possibly other amplifying hosts. Transmission of CHIKV occurs through a bite by infected *Ae. aegypti* or *Ae. albopictus*, although in the recent epidemic, some cases were the result of maternal–fetal transmission [12, 13, 18].

There is evidence that some animals, including non-primates, rodents, birds, and small mammals, may act as reservoirs of the virus, allowing re-emergence of the virus after periods of inactivity in humans [19].

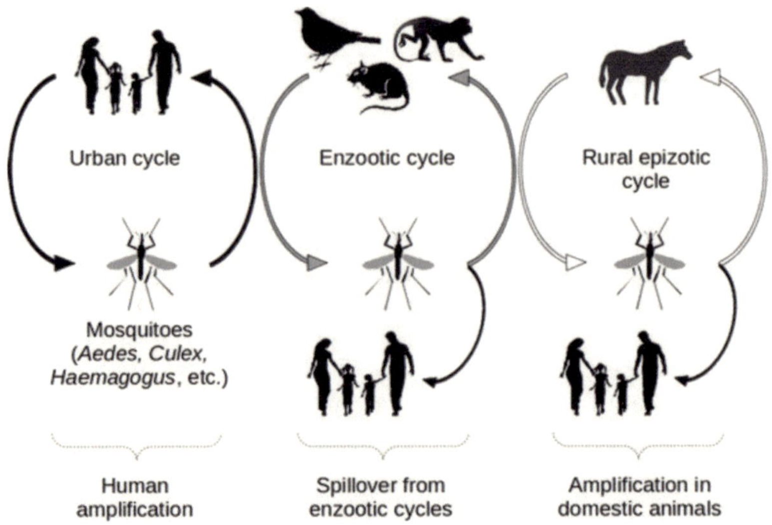

Figure 1.
Showing Chikungunya virus transmission cycles.

3.3 Mosquito-virus relationship

The ability of arthropods to transmit pathogens depends on intrinsic and extrinsic factors and is expressed in two terms: (a) Vector competence, the ability of a vector to become infected and transmit after the pathogen is ingested in a blood meal, is often regulated for arboviruses at the level of midgut infection, and (b) Vectorial capacity, the number of infective bites arising from an infected host, as shown in **Figure 2**. Host-seeking female mosquitoes are infected after feeding on a viremic animal. CHIKV first replicates in the midgut and then enters the hemocoel before disseminating to the salivary glands. Midgut basal lamina reorganization during blood digestion mediates this dissemination process. The extrinsic incubation period is generally 2–5 days, suggesting that even vector populations with poor daily adult survival can transmit effectively. Females with a disseminated virus in their salivary glands can transmit by injecting infectious saliva into a naïve host during a subsequent blood meal, leading to horizontal transmission. *Ae. aegypti* feeding is often interrupted when it is disturbed during blood feeding, and it may then complete the meal on one or more hosts in the vicinity. This can lead this

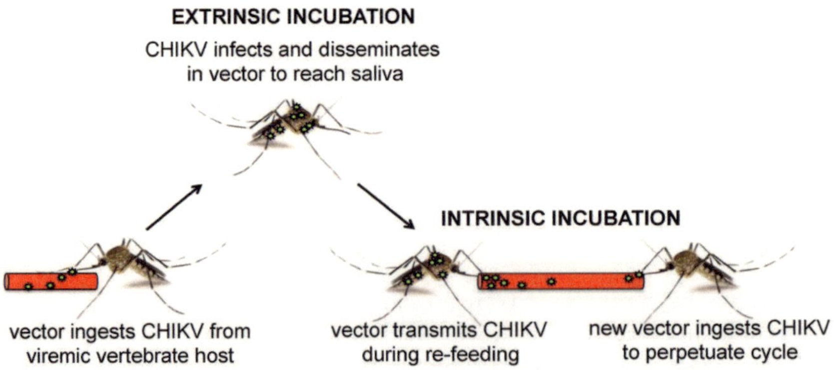

Figure 2.
Chikungunya virus in the host-vector transmission cycle.

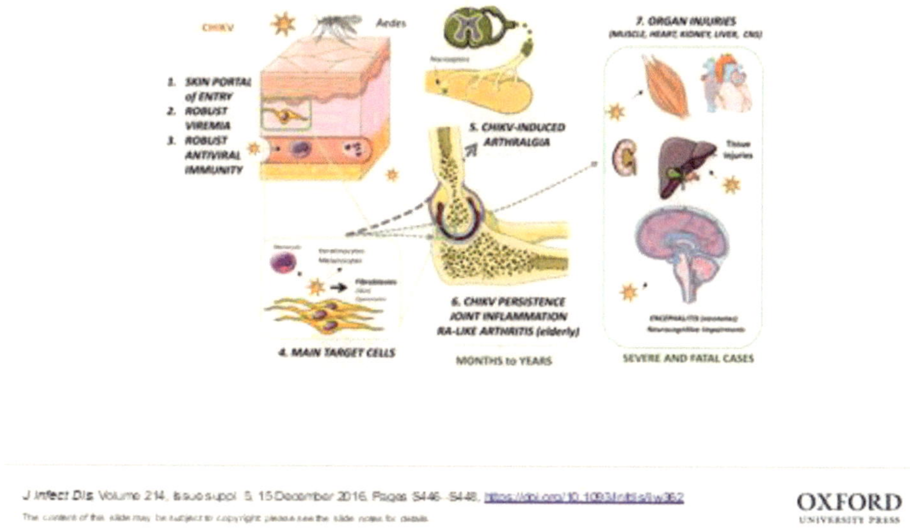

Figure 3.
Chikungunya pathogenesis.

highly anthropophilic species to feed on multiple persons daily, increasing the risk of CHIKV infection and transmission to multiple hosts, greatly enhancing vectorial capacity. Vector competence of *Ae. aegypti* and *Ae. albopictus* shows variation according to the geographical origin of the mosquito population and CHIKV strain [1, 15]. Once infectious, the mosquito is believed to be capable of transmitting the virus for the rest of its life.

3.4 Chikungunya pathogenesis

In order for the viral transmission to occur, the skin is a major portal of entry whereby the infested mosquito transmits CHIKV together with immunoregulatory proteins from the mosquito's saliva while taking a blood meal. The local immune response (monocyte, keratocytes, and melanocytes) cannot prevent the virus from spreading to other tissues. Then, CHIKV replicates in the fibroblast cells of the skin then through the blood circulation, the viruses are disseminated to the brain cells, the kidney, heart, lymphoid tissues, liver, and joints. The incubation period is 2–4 days and is followed by a sudden onset of clinical disease with no prodromal phase. Symptoms of CHIKV infection include high fever, rigors, headache, photophobia, and a petechial rash or maculopapular rash. In addition, most infected individuals complain of severe joint pain that is often incapacitating due to the joint inflammation caused by arthralgia and rheumatoid arthritis (**Figure 3**) [16, 20].

4. Recommendation

The use of a mosquito larvae management system would be a great approach to reduce vector population. The use of mosquito repellents, such as coils and lotions containing repellents, during the daytime will reduce arboviral transmissions. Governments could develop public awareness campaigns during outbreaks to educate populations on how to control the disease.

Author details

Lucille Lyaruu
Tropical Pesticides Research Institute, Arusha, Tanzania

*Address all correspondence to: lucillejustis@gmail.com

References

[1] Ganesan VK, Duan B, Reid SP. Chikungunya virus: Pathophysiology, mechanism, and modeling. Viruses. 2017;**9**:1-14. DOI: 10.3390/v9120368

[2] Braack L, Gouveia De Almeida AP, Cornel AJ, Swanepoel R, De Jager C. Mosquito-borne arboviruses of African origin: Review of key viruses and vectors. Parasites & Vectors. 2018;**11**. DOI: 10.1186/s13071-017-2559-9

[3] Hertz JT, Lyaruu LJ, Ooi EE, Mosha FW, Crump JA. Distribution of *Aedes* mosquitoes in the Kilimanjaro Region of Northern Tanzania. Pathogens and Global Health. 2016;**110**:108-112. DOI: 10.1080/20477724.2016.1182719

[4] Higa Y, Thi Yen N, Kawada H, Hai Son T, Thuy Hoa N, Takagi M. Geographic distribution of *Aedes aegypti* and *Aedes albopictus* collected from used tires in Vietnam. Journal of the American Mosquito Control Association. 2010;**26**:1-9. DOI: 10.2987/09-5945.1

[5] Katsuda Y, Leemingsawat S, Thongrungkiat S, Prummonkol S, Samung Y, Kanzaki T, et al. Control of mosquito vectors of tropical infectious diseases: (3) Susceptibility of *Aedes aegypti* to pyrethroid and mosquito coils. The Southeast Asian Journal of Tropical Medicine and Public Health. 2009;**40**

[6] Kamgang B, Ngoagouni C, Manirakiza A, Nakouné E, Paupy C, Kazanji M. Temporal patterns of abundance of *Aedes aegypti* and *Aedes albopictus* (Diptera: Culicidae) and mitochondrial DNA analysis of *Ae. albopictus* in the Central African Republic. PLoS Neglected Tropical Diseases. 2013;7. DOI: 10.1371/journal.pntd.0002590

[7] Kraemer MUG, Sinka ME, Duda KA, Mylne AQN, Shearer FM, Barker CM, et al. The global distribution of the arbovirus vectors *Aedes aegypti* and *Ae. albopictus*. eLife. 2015;**4**. DOI: 10.7554/eLife.08347

[8] Saleh F, Kitau J, Konradsen F, Alifrangis M, Lin C-H, Juma S, et al. Habitat characteristics for immature stages of *Aedes aegypti* in Zanzibar City, Tanzania. Journal of the American Mosquito Control Association. 2018;**34**:190-200. DOI: 10.2987/17-6709.1

[9] Steinwascher K. Competition among *Aedes aegypti* larvae. PLoS ONE. 2018;**13**. DOI: 10.1371/journal.pone.0202455

[10] Lacroix R, Delatte H, Hue T, Dehecq JS, Reiter P. Adaptation of the BG-Sentinel trap to capture male and female *Aedes albopictus* mosquitoes. Medical and Veterinary Entomology. 2009;**23**:160-162. DOI: 10.1111/j.1365-2915.2009.00806.x

[11] Chen Z, Liu F, Liu N. Human odour coding in the Yellow fever Mosquito, *Aedes aegypti*. Scientific Reports. 2019;**9**:13336. DOI: 10.1038/s41598-019-49753-2

[12] Smallegange R, Takken W. Host-seeking behaviour of mosquitoes: Responses to olfactory stimuli in the laboratory. Olfaction in Vector-Host Interactions. 2010:143-180

[13] Baraka V, Baraka V, Mathias L, Mathias L, Kweka J. We are IntechOpen, the world's leading publisher of Open Access books Built by scientists, for scientists TOP 1% n.d.

[14] Farjana T, Tuno N. Multiple blood feeding and host-seeking behavior in *Aedes aegypti* and *Aedes albopictus* (Diptera: Culicidae). Journal of Medical Entomology. 2013;**50**. DOI: 10.1603/ME12146

[15] Thiboutot MM, Kannan S, Kawalekar OU, Shedlock DJ, Khan AS, Sarangan G, et al. Chikungunya: A potentially emerging epidemic? PLoS Neglected Tropical Diseases. 2010;**4**:e623. DOI: 10.1371/journal.pntd.0000623

[16] Burt FJ, Rolph MS, Rulli NE, Mahalingam S, Heise MT. Chikungunya: A re-emerging virus. Lancet. 2012;**379**:662-671. DOI: 10.1016/S0140-6736(11)60281-X

[17] Saganda W, Munishi OM, Crump JA, Hertz JT, Howe S, Kinabo GD, et al. Chikungunya and dengue fever among hospitalized febrile patients in Northern Tanzania. The American Journal of Tropical Medicine and Hygiene. 2012;**86**:171-177. DOI: 10.4269/ajtmh.2012.11-0393

[18] Eastwood G, Sang RC, Guerbois M, Taracha ELN, Weaver SC. Enzootic circulation of Chikungunya virus in East Africa: Serological evidence in non-human Kenyan primates. The American Journal of Tropical Medicine and Hygiene. 2017;**97**:1399-1404. DOI: 10.4269/ajtmh.17-0126

[19] Kamgang B, Happi JY, Boisier P, Njiokou F, Hervé JP, Simard F, et al. Geographic and ecological distribution of the dengue and Chikungunya virus vectors *Aedes aegypti* and *Aedes albopictus* in three major Cameroonian towns. Medical and Veterinary Entomology. 2010;**24**:132-141. DOI: 10.1111/j.1365-2915.2010.00869.x

[20] Schwartz O, Albert ML. Biology and pathogenesis of Chikungunya virus. Nature Reviews. Microbiology. 2010;**8**:491-500. DOI: 10.1038/nrmicro2368

Section 5

Treatment and Prevention

Chapter 5

Treatment and Prevention of Chikungunya Fever: Current Status and Prospective

Merhawi Debesai Oqbazgi

Abstract

Chikungunya fever is a vector borne tropical disease that was first described in an outbreak in Tanzania. The disease is caused by Chikungunya virus (CHIKV), an alpha virus belonging to the family Togaviridae and which is transmitted from one person to another via the bite of mosquitoes. Active disease is characterized by high grade fever, pain and joint symptoms. Although debilitating at times, the disease seldom progresses to result in a serious outcome like death. There are no specific treatments for Chikungunya virus at the moment. Clinical case management is highly dependent on providing palliative care which in turn is expected to alleviate symptoms and accelerate recovery from the infection. An important element in the control of outbreaks of CHIKV infection is prevention. Preventive strategies involve initiatives like vector control, immunizations and extra care to patients with the infection. There have been several tens of researches focusing on the introduction of newer drugs and vaccines against Chikungunya. That being said, so far, no single agent has completed the entire drug or vaccine development process. Chikungunya fever is a neglected tropical disease. Although it has no specific treatment till date, the number of vaccine and drug candidates under study provides promising insights on the prospects on chikungunya treatment.

Keywords: Febrile Illnesses, Chikungunya Virus, Palliative Care and Vector Control

1. Introduction

Chikungunya fever was first described in Tanzania in the year 1952 during an outbreak in the southern part of the country. The disease is a vector borne infection transmitted by mosquitoes carrying the causative agent, Chikungunya virus (CHIKV), an RNA virus of the genus alphavirus and family Togaviridae [1]. CHIKV is transmitted to humans by bites of several species of mosquitoes, the two main species of mosquitoes transmitting the disease being *Aedes aegypti* and *Aedes albopictus* [2]. Major symptoms of the infection include fever (sudden high grade 39–40°C), muscle and joint pain, swelling (joints), headache, nausea and other minor skin reactions [3]. Deaths from severe infections are not common and if any, the deaths are usually linked to other underlying medical conditions. Persons suffering an active infection may develop debilitating joint pain that gives them a distinct curved or bent posture and this is from which the disease's name 'Chikungunya' was derived, which in the Makonde dialect means 'to be contorted or bent'.

Although Chikungunya fever occurs throughout the world, it is specifically common in the African continent. The disease is similar to many other febrile viral illnesses in terms of the clinical presentation of infected patients, thus; it can be misdiagnosed in areas where there are inadequacies of laboratory setups and testing procedures [4]. Even when it was first described as a disease in Tanzania, it was clinically indistinguishable from dengue fever [3]. For this reason, there are inaccuracies in the numbers of infections of Chikungunya reported from various setups and in many instances, it is almost impossible to come up with a reliable estimate of the prevalence of the infection.

Currently, there are no commercially available vaccines or any specific drugs to cure Chikungunya fever and existing treatments generally focus on relieving symptoms. That being said, there have been immense research throughout the years in pursuit of specific drug candidates and vaccines to target the causative agent, but yet; no single entity was made available to the world. The most effective intervention the world has been working on is to improve infection prevention strategies targeting activities ranging from vector control to prevention of mosquito bites and acquiring the infection.

This chapter provides brief highlights on the treatment approaches so far used, preventive strategies employed and promising prospective drug and vaccine candidates whose development have been underway in the past few years.

2. Management of Chikungunya fever

Management of any infectious disease generally requires meticulous examination and a differential diagnosis in order to ascertain what is being dealt with in the first place. Before starting to treat Chikungunya fever, it is of utmost importance to rule out other viral infections, like Zika virus and Dengue fever, that have similar clinical presentation. Although in its severe form Chikungunya is a debilitating illness, like all other viral illnesses, the viral load of CHIKV is lowered by the body's immune response, thus; the symptoms are self-limiting and patients usually fully recover.

There are generally two approaches into the treatment of any disease condition, namely the specific treatment that focuses on the cause of the disease and another is a non-specific intervention intended to alleviate symptoms of the disease. Today, there is no specific antiviral drug or vaccine intended for use against the CHIKV and for this reason, managing Chikungunya fever clinically is palliative, meaning it only focuses on relieving the symptoms [5]. There are various pharmacologic and non-pharmacologic approaches into doing this, the main of which are explored in the next section.

2.1 Symptomatic treatments

Symptomatic interventions generally work to alleviate the symptoms that may result from a disease condition without necessarily having to deal with the underlying cause of the disease itself. In case of Chikungunya, a number of pharmacologic and non-pharmacologic approaches may be used to alleviate symptoms of the febrile illness.

2.1.1 Non-pharmacologic palliative care

Non-pharmacologic interventions do not employ the use of active chemical entities that modify or make use of a specific biochemical and/or physiological processes to bring about the required change and thereby alleviate a symptom. Such interventions include life style elements like dietary modifications, fluid intake and bed rest. A common symptom in patients experiencing active Chikungunya infection is generalized body weakness and lethargy, thus; adequate nourishment and rest is very important to boost the patient's immune response. Consumption of citrus fruits and the use of multivitamin supplements may also be recommended in some cases where there is loss of appetite. Taking plenty of fluids on the other hand helps the patient to stay rehydrated thereby maintaining stamina and metabolic stability. All these interventions play a vital role in optimizing the immune attack the body launches against the virus and thus not only alleviate the symptoms, but also accelerate the whole recovery process.

2.1.2 Pharmacologic palliative care

Pharmacologic interventions employ the use of specific active pharmaceutical entities which make use of specific bodily biochemical and/or physiological pathways to bring about a specific effect and thereby alleviate a symptom. The most common symptoms namely fever and joint pain can be alleviated with the use of Non-Steroidal Anti-Inflammatory Drugs (NSAIDs). It is a fact that all NSAIDs have anti-pyretic (body temperature lowering) and analgesic (pain relieving) properties. Despite this fact, paracetamol or acetaminophen is more commonly used to manage fever and mild pain while drugs belonging to the same therapeutic class like ibuprofen, diclofenac and naproxen are used to alleviate pain to maintain a favorable risk–benefit balance when using those medicines. Although Aspirin belongs to the NSAIDs, its use for analgesia and as an anti-pyretic agent is not recommended. This is in particular because of its blood thinning properties, giving the drug an unfavorable risk–benefit balance when used for these specific indications.

There are a number of studies debating over the use of chloroquine to treat the arthritis like symptoms of Chikungunya fever. Even if there is evidence that chloroquine is effective in managing various rheumatic joint diseases, its use for the management of Chikungunya fever related joint symptoms remains questionable. Disease-modifying anti-rheumatic drugs are also claimed to be effective in treating Chikungunya virus induced symptoms of chronic joint diseases that resemble rheumatoid arthritis in their presentation. The literature also presents other medicines like eupatorium perf, influenzinum, rhus-tox, pyroginum and cedron that are primarily utilized in south east Asia and are believed to play curative and preventive roles.

Interventions to alleviate symptoms of Chikungunya, whether non-pharmacologically or pharmacologically, are believed to be effective in improving prognosis and overall accelerating full recovery form the illness. A careful consideration should however be made when selecting an appropriate treatment, particularly a pharmacological palliative intervention, for the patient so that the risk benefit balance of using the treatment remains favorable.

2.2 Specific treatments

In principle, a specific treatment is supposed to completely cure a disease. This would mean that the treatment will precisely target the pathophysiological root cause of the disease in the case of non-infectious disease and the invading causative agent in the case of an infectious disease.

Till date, there is no single antiviral entity proven to be specifically effective against the CHIKV. There have however been several antiviral candidates under study to target the virus. With regard to active and passive immunizations against

Approach	Specific intervention	Example:
Palliative care	Non-pharmacologic treatment	**Real-time:** Dietary modification, rehydration and bed rest all play key role in boosting the immune responses against the virus and thus facilitating full recovery.
	Pharmacologic treatment	**Real-time:** The use of NSAIDs such as paracetamol or ibuprofen to alleviate fever and indomethacin or diclofenac to relieve joint pain.
Specific treatment	Antiviral drugs	**Prospective:** Specific antiviral drugs that target CHIKV by interfering with the various vital steps in the viral replication cycle such as attachment, penetration, un-coating, replication, assembly, and release.
	Therapeutic (passive) immunization	**Prospective:** The use of specific preformed antibodies that directly target the whole virus or viral coat molecules there by clearing viral particles.

Table 1.
Real-time and prospective approaches for the management of chikungunya fever.

the virus, no vaccine is commercially available for use in humans today. There are however several vaccine strategies under study and some vaccine candidates have now reached to advanced stages in the clinical development process. These candidates are however still long way from the approval step and longer way from being available in markets for consumption.

The management of Chikungunya fever is primarily palliative. Until the time when specific curative alternatives are made available, it is recommended that health practitioners make wise use of the available treatment options. Moreover, there are various recommended treatment guidelines specific to Chikungunya fever that provide clear steps on how effectively one can manage the infection [3].

Table 1 summarizes the various approaches used today and the likely to be future treatment options in the management of CHIKV.

3. Preventive measures

The prevention of disease acquirement and transmission is key to halt the spread of any infectious disease. In case of Chikungunya virus infection, prevention becomes vital to control spread especially that there are no specific treatments against the disease. There may be several preventive strategies to control the spread of Chikungunya fever. For the purpose of clarity, this section summarizes them into three major approaches namely vector control measures, immunizations and care for the already diseased persons.

3.1 Vector control and avoiding mosquito bites

Chikungunya is an arthropod borne viral infection. CHIKV is transmitted to humans by bites of several species of mosquitoes [2, 3]. The two main species of mosquitoes transmitting the disease are *Aedes aegypti* and *Aedes albopictus*. *Aedes aegypti* is commonly responsible for transmission in urban areas whereas *Aedes albopictus* has been the main vector in rural areas. These mosquitoes can be easily distinguishable from others by the presence of white markings on their limbs and a marking in the form of a lyre on the upper surface of the thorax. Recognizing the mosquito itself is very important as it gives an insight into the possibility of the existence of an outbreak in a specific area.

The control and termination of breeding of the vector is key to the prevention of the transmission of any vector borne infection. In the control of CHIKV outbreaks, vector control through the use of larvicides and adulticides, the removal of larval habitats, limiting human-vector contact and public education is critical [6]. The measures that should be taken in vector control are similar to those used in the control of transmission of malaria. The common measures that should be taken include:

- Emptying and scrubbing, turning over, burying, covering, or throwing out items that hold water. Since mosquitoes need water to lay eggs, it is very important to cover or dry swampy spots in the surrounding of the outdoors of living places.

- Using insecticides and repellents to kill and/or keep away mosquitoes from indoors and thereby avoiding bites.

Another important measure that should be taken to control the spread of CHIKV is to avoid mosquito bites. There are a few things that can be done to avoid bites:

- Recognizing the mosquito based on its physical appearance (white markings) and being aware that unlike the mosquitoes that spread malaria which are usually active and bite during the night time, the Aedes species are active and bite during both the day and the night times.

- Sleeping under a mosquito net especially in areas where mosquito breeding rates are very high. Such places may include high humidity and swampy areas.

- Applying mosquito repellents. There are a wide variety of products that contain mosquito repellents and are available in different formulations such as lotions and creams.

Since mosquitoes have a major role in the spread of CHIKV, targeting them is key to halt the transmission cycle. Vector control comprises a set of activities, not limited to the above described, intended to minimize transmission of CHIKV and thereby the occurrence of active Chikungunya infections.

3.2 Immunization

Active immunization against specific foreign entities entering the human body has been one of the most effective strategies in the prevention of communicable diseases. Like other infectious diseases, CHIKV has been a subject of interest for many vaccine developers. There is however no vaccine that have been made commercially available for preventive immunizations against the disease.

Recent studies list a number of candidates that are under development [7, 8]. Of the candidates, there is a single vaccine that have made progress to phase three clinical trials, which seems to be the most progressing out of the rest of the candidates [9]. That being said, according to what is published in the scientific literature thus far, making a vaccine available for human use does not seem to be something that one should expect in the very near future.

S.No.	Strategy	Category	Description
1.	Vector Control	Minimizing mosquito breeding	Controlling mosquito habitats (water holes, swamps and dump areas) and use of insecticides, larvicides and adulticides to limit vector proliferation.
		Avoiding mosquito bites	Sleeping under mosquito nets, avoiding shorts and short sleeved wears during both day and night times (to minimize open exposure of the skin surface) and the application of mosquito repellents.
2.	Immunizations	Active immunization	Vaccinating healthy individuals to develop active immunity against the infection. With no consideration given to their safety profile, only a few vaccine candidates have shown demonstrable efficacy in eliciting adequate immune responses against CHIKV.
3.	Patient care	Host control	Infected patients are sources of the virus. Protecting the infected patient from further mosquito bites reduces the chances of transmission.
4.	Health education	Public awareness	Educating the public on the preventive strategies and how to seek medical care if they suspect they are infected. Moreover, describing the mosquito, its physical features and behavior.

Table 2.
Strategies for the prevention of spread of CHIKV.

3.3 Special care for the diseased

Just as the mosquito plays a major role in the transmission cycle of CHIKV, so does the infected patient. The already diseased patient is actually incubating the causative agent. It is, for this very reason, important that infected persons be protected from further mosquito exposure during the first few days of the illness when the viral load is high, so they can not contribute to the transmission cycle. Preventing further mosquito bites can be achieved through the same measures listed under the vector control and bite prevention strategies.

The main preventive strategies that could be adopted to limit outbreaks of CHIKV are briefly described in **Table 2**.

The world has not gone too far in developing a specific cure for Chikungunya fever. Apart from the common notion that 'prevention is better than cure', in the case of Chikungunya, prevention becomes of a particular interest because, until today, there are no specific antiviral therapies or vaccines (whether active or passive immunizations) that are proven to be safe and effective. It is hence important that centers of disease control and prevention pay due attention in this regard and take proactive measures to prevent or at least limit outbreaks.

4. Prospects on the introduction of new drugs and vaccines

As is the case with many other bacterial, viral or fungal infectious diseases, Chikungunya fever has been a subject of interest for many researchers in pursuit of new drug therapies and vaccines. Despite the fact that much effort has been done so far, there is still no antiviral proven to be specifically effective against CHIKV while being safe for use in humans [10]. Moreover, no vaccine has been made available for use by humans. It is however worth reflecting the trends on the development of newer drugs and vaccines for chikungunya and to explore the various strategies employed in their development. This particular section summarizes the prospects in drug and vaccine development for Chikungunya fever.

4.1 Development of antiviral agents and the strategies employed

An antiviral agent is an entity that specifically targets a virus resulting in disruption of viral particles, prevention of replication and/or acceleration of viral clearance through immunological mechanisms.

There have been a number of trails conducted in pursuit of a safe and effective antiviral agents working specifically against the CHIKV. The candidates being tested in the different trials are variable and target CHIKV through variable ways. Some of the agents under study are small CHIKV inhibitor molecules and others are natural inhibitors of viral replication [8, 11]. There are also repurposed drugs, monoclonal antibodies, gene silencers and viral particles that work more or less through immune modulation. In the last decade, more than 30 antiviral agents that are thought to be effective against CHIKV were patented [8]. There are several antiviral agents studied so far, the description of some of which is briefly explored below.

4.1.1 Inhibitors of CHIKV

The CHIKV inhibitors is a category comprising a large array of compounds including small inhibitor molecules, inhibitors from natural sources, repurposed drugs and so on. This drugs utilize various biochemical pathways to inhibit the replication of CHIKV. There are several tens of agents being studied under this category, the majority of which are in the early stages of drug development. For instance, ribavirin, arbidol, chloroquine, Epigallocatechin Gallate (EGCG) and ribostamycin sulfate are some of the many drugs that fall under this category [8].

CHIKV inhibitors exert their antiviral actions through a number of mechanisms. Majority of these agents are viral replication inhibitors. They interfere in various stages of viral replication such as gene transcription, assembly of viral particles into virions and budding of virions out from the host cell. Other agents are thought to contribute to viral clearance by the immune responses. None of these agents has fully gone through the entire drug development process and thus non are made available in the market.

4.1.2 Monoclonal antibodies

The use of monoclonal antibodies in the treatment of various infectious and non-infectious diseases has been a very helpful strategy in the past few decades. Monoclonal antibodies are more or less a simple model of passive immunizations where preformed antibodies work to directly infiltrate viral particles.

There are many trials made on agents being developed as monoclonal antibodies to work against CHIKV. The introduction of antibodies that are effective against proteins of CHIKV could be a potential approach leading to vaccine development as a treatment. These agents that make use of the immune system of the host stimulates various immune modulators such as type I interferons and antibodies during the initial stages of an infection with CHIKV [12], Immunoglobulin M (IgM) antibodies during an acute phase [13] and Immunoglobulin G (IgG) antibodies for infections persisting longer [14]. Neutralizing antibodies can be of help to prevent budding of CHIKV from infected host cells and thus interfere with the viral release from the host stage of the replication process [15].

In this prospect, the use of Monoclonal antibodies seems to be a very promising approach towards the introduction of new antiviral treatments against Chikungunya in the not too far future.

4.1.3 Vaccines

Although generally and in principle vaccines have a bigger role in the prevention of acquiring active diseases, their use as therapeutic agents have become a commonly employed strategy especially in the essence of passive immunization where recipients are given readily made antibodies that directly work to neutralize the causative agent. The previously discussed principle about monoclonal antibodies was more or less preceded by such ideas about neutralization.

In the area of vaccine development against Chikungunya, various efforts have been made in the last decade to develop effective vaccines for the treatment of CHIKV infections. A number of live-attenuated virus vaccines, inactivated virus vaccine, recombinant viral component vaccines, DNA and mRNA-based vaccines, synthetic vaccines, subunit formulations of CHIKV and others have been developed [16]. Further details on vaccine development will be discussed in the section that follows.

4.2 Development of vaccines and the strategies employed

The introduction of vaccinations against CHIKV has been a subject of interest ever since the disease was first described decades back. Immunizations in general can be active and/or passive. Active immunization refers to the exposure of the body to a foreign entity resulting in the initiation of body's immune responses weather cell mediated or antibody mediated. The development of immunological memory will then result in prompt immune responses in subsequent invasions by the foreign agent to which memory was developed. On the other hand, passive immunization refers to the transfer, into the body, of readily made antibodies that may directly act upon the foreign entity in the body. In this case, the neutralization of the invading agent is much faster as there is no time lapse between sensitization and secretion of antibodies. In the development of vaccines against chikungunya, both types of vaccine agents have been under study [17].

4.2.1 Passive immunization

Passive immunization against the CHIKV refers to the introduction of preformed antibodies that directly act upon the causative virus. This is briefly discussed in the previous section where monoclonal antibodies are presented as therapeutic antiviral agents. Human protection from CHIKV infection is primarily mediated by humoral memory host response and the presence of neutralizing antibodies targeting the virus's outer surfaces of envelope glycoproteins [18]. There are studies that support the efficacy of monoclonal antibodies as post exposure therapy against CHIKV infections. Passive immunization therefore seems to be another prospect for the introduction of effective interventions against chikungunya in the future.

4.2.2 Active immunization

Active immunization employs the introduction of an antigen into the body to elicit an immune response and memory against the foreign agent. It is considered to be the most cost-effective preventive health intervention so far. The development of

Entity	Category	Description
Antiviral agent	Inhibitors of CHIKV (simple molecules)	• A group of compounds that interfere with various steps in the viral replication cycle. • More than 30 candidates under study. • Example: ribavirin and arbidol.
	Monoclonal antibodies	• Target specific immune modulators that neutralize virions. • Example: monoclonal antibodies that stimulate immune response mediators such as type I interferons, IgM and IgG in various stages of the infection.
Vaccine	Passive immunization	• Preformed antibodies that directly act to clear virions. • Fast onset of action (neutralization). • Example: serum purified antibodies.
	Active immunization	• Antigen based antibodies that stimulate the immune system to develop memory against CHIKV. • Example: vaccine candidates under development such as VRC-CHKV133, MVCHIK127 and CHIKV/IRES115.

Table 3.
CHIKV drug and vaccine development strategies.

a CHIKV vaccine seems to be feasible because the virus has a relatively low antigen diversity compared to other similar viruses [17]. This would also imply that changes in vaccine effectiveness profiles, assuming an effective vaccine is made available, are less likely to occur due to the less rapid rate of mutations observed with the virus.

Until 2016, three experimental vaccines have advanced to the stage of human testing. Two candidates namely, the VRC-CHKV133 and the MVCHIK127 vaccines finished phase I, in 2014 and 2015 respectively. The third candidate (CHIKV/IRES115 vaccine) yielded promising efficacy and safety results in mice and macaques and plans are in place for a phase I trial. It is worth of note that there is one candidate that have advanced to phase three trials in 2020 [9]. This prospect gave hope to many disease control program managers.

Table 3 provides a summary list of the most advancing drug and vaccine development approaches for CHIKV.

5. Chapter summary

Chikungunya fever is a vector borne infection caused by Chikungunya virus. The virus is transmitted by the bites of two main mosquito species namely, *Aedes aegypti* and *Aedes albopictus*. The disease is characterized by several symptoms the major of which are high grade fever, joint pain and joint inflammation. Severe infections are debilitating and may require the patient to be bedbound or may even result in death, though very rare, in cases where the patient has a compromised overall health status.

Currently, there are no specific anti-viral drugs against the Chikungunya virus and treatments are designed to alleviate symptoms. There are a number of palliative pharmacological and non-pharmacological treatment options which may offer symptomatic relief and accelerate recovery from the infection. The use of non-steroidal anti-inflammatory agents to alleviate fever, pain and various joint symptoms associated with the disease has been a very effective management option. Some other non-medicinal life style approaches like dietary changes such as consumption of more vitamins and minerals to boost the immune response to the infection have also been some of the recommended care approaches. The overall goal of palliative care is to reduce suffering and accelerate recovery.

Exploring the various preventive strategies adopted to minimize the transmission of Chikungunya virus is of utmost importance. The general notion of disease prevention is more pronounced when treatment options are limited or inexistent. The absence of specific treatment for Chikungunya therefore necessitates that due attention is given to prevention. Although several strategies may be employed to prevent viral transmission, vector control has been the one major approach to halt spread of the infection. Prevention of mosquito bites becomes as important to the already infected as it is for the uninfected person in terminating the transmission cycle. In another scene, despite the recognition that immunizations have for so long been the most cost effective preventive health interventions and the efforts made to discover some, no specific CHIKV vaccine has so far been made commercially available and thus the use of vaccines as preventive measures is yet to come.

As it is the case with many novel viral diseases, Chikungunya has for decades been a subject of interest to drug and vaccine development firms. The current status and prospective with regard to new drug and vaccine development and clinical trials for cures and immunizations against this viral disease seems to be promising. Many new trails on animal models are currently underway and a few drug and vaccine candidates made it to testing in humans. Several tens of antiviral agents have advanced to the late stages of drug development. These entities come in various forms ranging from simple molecules, agents from natural sources and macromolecules such as monoclonal antibodies. On the other hand, a number of vaccines have also been under development and one candidate has so far advanced to phase three clinical trials, thus demonstrating acceptable safety and efficacy.

In light of the seriousness and debilitating nature of Chikungunya fever, the pursuit for newer treatment options and preventive strategies such as vaccinations should inevitably be encouraged. Neglected tropical diseases, as their name implies, have for long been ignored in many aspects in attempts to favor policies and resource allocations towards diseases that are deemed deserving priority based on their public health threat profile. Chikungunya fever is a neglected tropical disease, yet, the bulk of research carried out in this area is commendable and the trends demonstrate a possibility for the introduction of a novel treatment option in the near future.

Acknowledgements

This book chapter was prepared by conducting a through literature review and no source of funding was used to prepare the manuscript.

Declaration

Conflict of Interest: The author declares that he has no competing interests.

Funding: No funding was solicited for the preparation of this chapter.

Consent for Publication: The author gives his consent for publication.

Ethical clearance/approval: This is a book chapter not a research article employing subjects of study and thus, no ethical clearance was sought (not applicable).

Data or Information privacy policy: To the author's awareness, no data set was used in contrary to terms of data privacy policy and/or intellectual property rights in the preparation of this chapter. Specific factual information is well referenced.

Author details

Merhawi Debesai Oqbazgi
National Medicines and Food Administration, Ministry of Health, Asmara, Eritrea

*Address all correspondence to: dome.bable07@gmail.com

References

[1] World Health Organization (WHO). Chikungunya fever factsheet 2020 [Updated September 15, 2020]. Available from: https://www.who.int/news-room/fact-sheets/detail/chikungunya.

[2] Centers for Disease Control and Prevention, National Center for Emerging and Zoonotic Infectious Diseases (NCEZID), Division of Vector-Borne Diseases (DVBD). Chikungunya prevention 2020 [Updated December 07, 2020]. Available from: https://www.cdc.gov/chikungunya/index.html.

[3] World Health Organization (WHO). Guidelines on clinical management of chikungunya fever. WHO Regional Office for South-East Asia, 2008.

[4] Soto-Garita C, Carrera J-P, López-Vergès S, Corrales-Aguilar E. Advances in clinical diagnosis and Management of Chikungunya Virus Infection. Current Treatment Options in Infectious Diseases. 2018;10(3):397-409.

[5] Subudhi BB, Chattopadhyay S, Mishra P, Kumar A. Current strategies for inhibition of chikungunya infection. Viruses. 2018;10(5):235.

[6] CDC. CHIKUNGUNYA information for vector control programs 2015 [Updated July 9, 2015]. Available from: http://www.cdc.gov/chikungunya/pdfs/CHIKV_VectorControl.pdf

[7] An W, Ge N, Cao Y, Sun J, Jin X. Recent progress on chikungunya virus research. Virologica Sinica. 2017;32(6):441-453.

[8] Ghildiyal R, Gabrani R. Antiviral therapeutics for chikungunya virus. Expert opinion on therapeutic patents. 2020;30(6):467-480.

[9] Carlson R. Chikungunya vaccine candidate heads to phase 3 study: Valneva chikungunya vaccine candidate VLA1553 reduces clinical illness risk. Precision Vaccinations. 2020.

[10] Tharmarajah K, Mahalingam S, Zaid A. Chikungunya: vaccines and therapeutics. F1000Research. 2017;6.

[11] Parashar D, Cherian S. Antiviral perspectives for chikungunya virus. BioMed Research International. 2014;2014.

[12] Fox JM, Diamond MS. Immune-mediated protection and pathogenesis of chikungunya virus. The Journal of Immunology. 2016;197(11):4210-4218.

[13] Broeckel R, Fox JM, Haese N, Kreklywich CN, Sukulpovi-Petty S, Legasse A, et al. Therapeutic administration of a recombinant human monoclonal antibody reduces the severity of chikungunya virus disease in rhesus macaques. PLoS neglected tropical diseases. 2017;11(6):e0005637.

[14] Kam Y-W, Lee WW, Simarmata D, Harjanto S, Teng T-S, Tolou H, et al. Longitudinal analysis of the human antibody response to chikungunya virus infection: Implications for serodiagnosis and vaccine development. Journal of virology. 2012;86(23):13005-13015.

[15] Jin J, Galaz-Montoya JG, Sherman MB, Sun SY, Goldsmith CS, O'Toole ET, et al. Neutralizing antibodies inhibit chikungunya virus budding at the plasma membrane. Cell host & microbe. 2018;24(3):417-28. e5.

[16] Cimica V, Galarza JM. Adjuvant formulations for virus-like particle (VLP) based vaccines. Clinical Immunology. 2017;183:99-108.

[17] Schwameis M, Buchtele N, Wadowski PP, Schoergenhofer C, Jilma B. Chikungunya vaccines in development. Human vaccines & immunotherapeutics. 2016;12(3): 716-731.

[18] Fong RH, Banik SS, Mattia K, Barnes T, Tucker D, Liss N, et al. Exposure of epitope residues on the outer face of the chikungunya virus envelope trimer determines antibody neutralizing efficacy. Journal of virology. 2014;88(24):14364-14379.

Chapter 6

Treatment of Chikungunya Virus (CHIKV) Using Targeted Immunotherapy

Fleury Augustin Nsole Biteghe,
Chalomie Nyangone Ekome Toung, Jean De La Croix Ndong,
Neelakshi Mungra, Tahir B. Dar and Arnaud John Kombe Kombe

Abstract

Chikungunya virus (CHIKV) is the most common mosquito-borne *Alphavirus* infecting humans worldwide. Up to date, there are no antiviral treatments or vaccines approved to treat or prevent CHIKV for which treatments remain symptomatic based on clinical manifestations. Hence, designing effective therapies to either prevent or treat CHIKV infection is of paramount importance. Interestingly, monoclonal antibodies (mAbs) are known to be significantly important in mediating protective immunity in CHIV infection. During the last decades, numerous animal studies have reported the protective and prophylactic efficacy of human and mouse anti-CHIKV mAbs isolated from convalescent patients. However, the therapeutic benefits of these anti-CHIKV mAbs can be limited by multiple factors. Thus, it becomes pertinent to better understand the CHIKV infection dynamics, mitigate the undesired mAbs-associated effects and improve therapies. In this review, we critically discuss CHIKV antiviral infectious mechanisms and address how the improved understanding of the latter may pave the way to better targeted immunotherapies.

Keywords: Therapeutics, Antibodies, Vaccines, Prophylactics, Chikungunya virus

1. Introduction

Chikungunya virus (CHIKV) is an arthropod-borne virus firstly discovered during the Tanzanian outbreak in 1952 and isolated a year later (1953) from patient serum and mosquitoes [1]. CHIKV is a worldwide epidemic threat responsible for self-limited fever, maculopapular rashes, and debilitating polyarthralgia in most (90–92%) infected patients [1, 2]. Its name, meaning "that which contorts or bends up" in "Kimakonde", a Tanzanian and Mozambican vernacular language, stems from the stooped posture exhibited by infected patients [3–6]. In endemic areas, CHIKV can be misdiagnosed as it displays dengue (DENV) or zika virus (ZIKV) like symptoms [1, 7]. Although less lethal, CHIKV-associated mortality rate can be influenced by other factors, including immunocompromised individuals, newborns from high viremic mothers or patients with preexisting arthritis [1]. CHIKV represents a serious economic burden, affecting the physical status of infected patients, restraining them from working for up to 35 days, as reported during the 2007 Indian outbreak [8]. For that reason, CHIKV was categorized as a biodefense pathogen by the National Institute of Allergy and Infectious Diseases (NIAID) in the USA [9]. Presently, there are no clinically licensed vaccines or therapies to treat CHIKV. Nonetheless, several pre-clinical animal models using antibody-based immunotherapy have shown some promising results in preventing and treating CHIKV infections [1, 7, 9, 10]. Despite several obstacles that have to be overcome to reach clinical fruition of such therapy [11], mAbs therapies offer better therapeutic avenues with respect to emerging disease outbreaks [12]. Hence, this review succinctly describes CHIKV characteristics (Transmission, structure and diagnosis) and highlights the potential therapeutic usage of mAbs based on their protective role in naturally occurring humoral immunity following CHIV infection. Lastly, we briefly discuss some challenges associated with mAbs therapy and propose future alternative therapeutic approaches.

2. Chikungunya's transmission cycle

CHIKV can be transmitted either horizontally from human to human through mosquito bites (*Aedes* species) [1] or vertically from a mother to a child during pregnancy or at birth, thus causing severe neonatal infection [1, 13, 14]. However, the rate of CHIKV transmission can be affected by the geographical location and the vector. It has been historically reported that CHIKV was predominant in Sub-Saharan Africa (SSA), Southeast Asia tropical and sub-tropical regions, where two different transmission cycles occur [15]. In rural areas, CHIKV replicates through a sylvatic transmission cycle (animal to human transmission via the mosquito), involving forest or savanna *Aedes* mosquitoes (*A. furcifer and A. africanus*) and animals (domestics and non-domestics), representing the main CHIKV reservoirs within this cycle [16]. The urban transmission cycle is mediated by *A. albopictus* (also known as Asian tiger mosquito) and *A. aegypti*, both maintaining the human-to-human transmission, thus making humans the principal CHIKV reservoirs in the urban epidemic cycle (**Figure 1**). Interestingly, Chikungunya fever outbreaks in Asia have been associated with only the

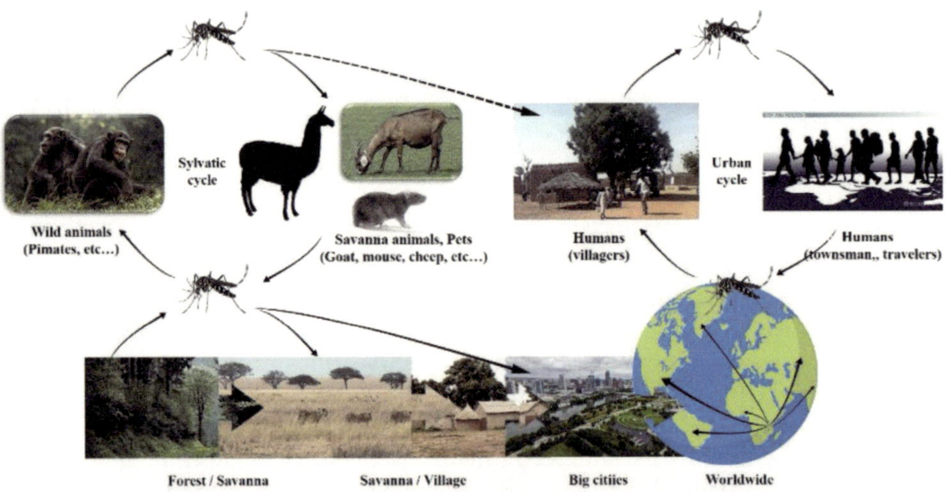

Figure 1.
CHIKV transmission cycle: Two cycles known as sylvatic and urban characterized the CHIKV transmission cycle. While the sylvatic predominantly occurs in Africa and circulates between primates, rodents and other vertebrates, the urban counterparts is commonly observed in Asia, where CHIKV is horizontally transferred from human to human through mosquito bites or blood meal.

urban CHIKV transmission cycle, while the African counterparts are related to both sylvatic and urban transmission cycles [15, 17]. Based on this evidence, it can hypothetically be suggested that the CHIKV transmission cycle before 1952 was restricted to the sylvatic cycle and that its urban transmission resulted from demographic expansion through deforestation or migration of CHIKV infected travelers from rural to the most populated urban cities. While the natural factors sustaining CHIKV infection remain elusive [16], it can be hypothesized that simultaneous presence of *Aedes* specie mosquitoes and CHIKV carriers (even with very low viral load in the blood) in a given area is enough for the resurgence of CHIKV-associated outbreaks.

3. Clinical manifestations of chikungunya fever

Chikungunya virus (CHIKV) is an emerging and re-emerging arbovirus associated with high morbidity, characterized by multiple clinical symptoms, with typical and/or atypical signs. CHIKV infection can be broken down into three phases, including the acute (the first 21st days following the onset of clinical symptoms), post-acute (from the 3rd week till the end of the 3rd month) and chronic phase (3 months following the onset of clinical symptoms) [1]. Therefore, chikungunya can present diverse clinical symptoms, for which 3–25% of infected individuals are asymptomatic (**Figure 2**) [18]. During the symptomatic phase, the majority of infected patients (90–95%) develop long lasting clinical symptoms coinciding with viremia peak (Elevated viral load ranging between 10^5 and 10^{12} viruses per milliliter of blood) and manifested as debilitating polyarthralgia, myalgia and arthralgia which are rarely fatal (1 in 1000) and not observed in dengue fever [18–20]. Atypical cases of CHIKV occur less frequently and mainly affect elderly, immunocompromised individuals and neonates from viremic mothers [1, 18]. The clinical manifestations associated with these atypical cases include severe neurological dysfunctions (Encephalitis), ocular changes, cardiovascular defect, preterm birth, hyperpigmentation, bullous dermatosis and Guillain-Barré syndrome [1, 18].

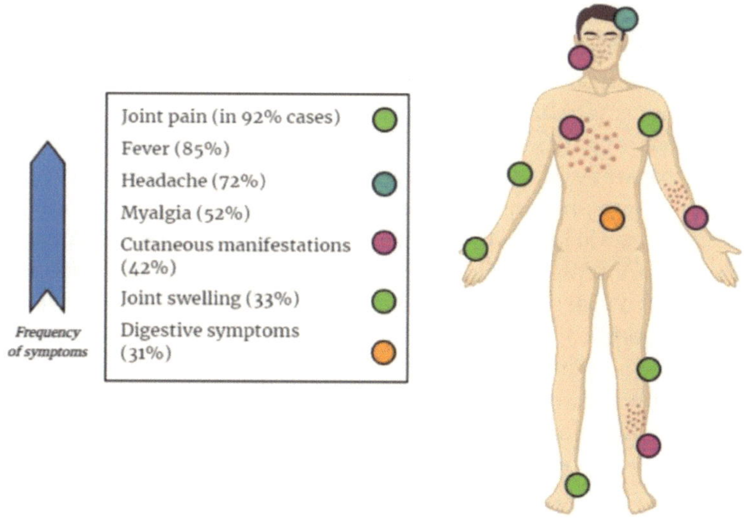

Figure 2.
Acute CHIKV clinical symptoms: During the symptomatic phase, CHIKV reportedly causes self-limited fever, as well as debilitating polyarthralgia in most (85–92%) infected patients [18–20]. Also, CHIKV can manifest atypical dermatological symptoms (42%) including edema, hemorrhagic bullous skin lesions, hyperpigmentation [21] and neurological symptoms, characterized by encephalopathy, encephalitis, Guillain-Barre or encephalomyelora-diculitis [22].

Yet, the mechanisms contributing to the long-lasting clinical symptoms remain elusive. An attempt to elucidate this mechanism was made by Reddy et al., 2017, demonstrating CHIKV's ability to evade host immunity as a result of CHIKV E1 glycoprotein homology to the host human counterpart [23]. Consequently, a more detailed understanding of CHIKV replication and infectious cycle is necessary to mitigate these undesired effects.

4. Chikungunya virus genome structure and infectious cycle

CHIKV is a small enveloped virus with a positive single-strand RNA virus belonging to the *Alphavirus* genus from the *Togaviridae* family [1, 21]. It is also referred to as an arbovirus (for *ar*thropod-*bo*rne *virus*) due to arthropods transmission (*Aedes* mosquitoes) [21]. CHIKV has an RNA genome of approximately 11.8 kb, comprising two open reading frames (ORFs), known as 5'caped ORF (7424 nucleotides) and 3'polyadenylated ORF (3732 nucleotides), linked by a junction region [22]. The 5'end is protected by a 7-methylguanosine (7MG) cap, with the ORF accounting for 66% of the genome encoding a precursor protein, which upon processing produces four nonstructural proteins (nsP1–4) responsible for CHIKV replication in host cell cytoplasm upon entry [1, 22]. On the other hand, the 3'ORF ends with a polyadenylation signal (3'poly-A tail) and encodes another precursor protein, generating five structural polyprotein comprising: the capsid C, envelop glycoproteins (E1, E2 and E3) and the 6 K protein [1, 22]. **Figure 3A** give a graphic representation of CHIKV genome. Once matured (after replicating in host cells), the virion particle has about 70 nm diameter and possesses 240 copies of capsid proteins embedded in 80 spikes of envelope trimers (glycoproteins E2/E1), which are inserted within the plasma membrane of the infected cells (to evade host immunity) that they use to bud out of the host cells through a secretory pathway [1, 22] (**Figure 3B**). Therefore, elucidating CHIKV replication cycle in both mammalian and mosquito cells becomes pertinent to develop efficient therapies.

CHIKV primarily replicates in the epithelial cells of mosquito midgut before migrating into the salivary glands where they keep replicating throughout the insect life, prior dissemination into the bloodstream of mammalian host, following mosquito bite/blood meal [1, 25]. Once deposited in the human bloodstream or skin after an infected mosquito bite (or blood meal), CHIKV firstly replicates within fibroblasts and macrophages found at the site of inoculation [16]. Thereafter, CHIKV systemically propagates within the body through the lymphatic system to multiple replication sites, where prominent disease symptoms occur (lymph nodes, spleen, skin, muscles, peripheral joints, brain, liver and tendons) despite innate immunity [16]. Notably, CHIKV replication in peripheral tissues is associated with elevated viral loads ($>10^9$ virus particles/ml), which is conducive for mosquito transmission during episodic bloodmeal or bite [16, 26]. Moreover, CHIKV can be transmitted to humans in various ways, including infected needles, contaminated blood donation, organ graft and from viremic mother to newborn [1, 27]. In this regard, Campos et al., 2017 study primarily highlighted the presence of CHIKV in the breast milk of an infected mother, who tested positive for serum and urine [28]. Fortunately, this study did not reveal a breastfeeding transmission capacity of the infected breast milk, as the 3-month-old newborn CHIKV serology and reverse transcriptase-polymerase chain reaction (RT-PCR) tested negative [1, 28]. In light of the latter results, it is worth mentioning that only the structural proteins (surface glycoproteins E2 and E1) are present on the outer surface of CHIKV envelop and are endowed with antigenic potential, able to elicit activation of host immune defense mechanisms [10].

(A)

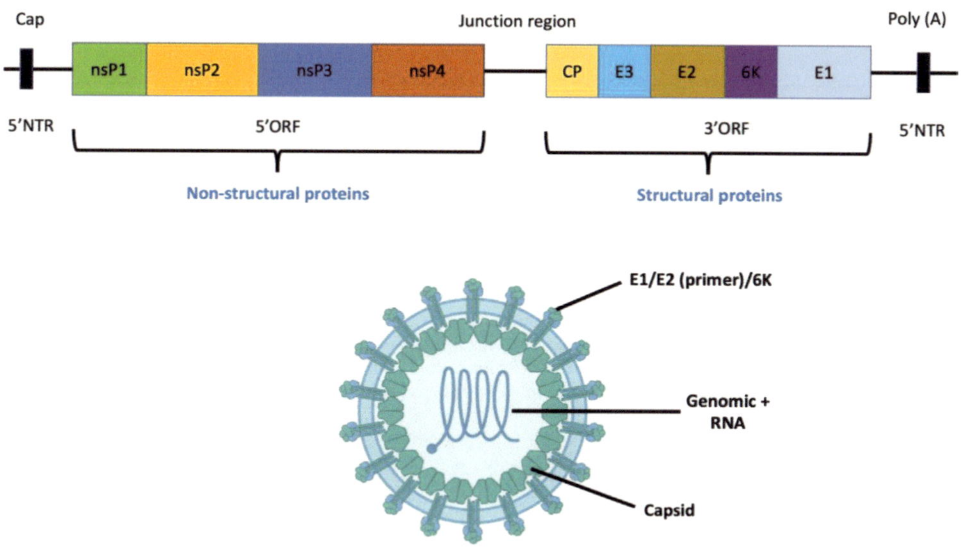
Cap
Junction region
Poly (A)
nsP1
nsP2
nsP3
nsP4
CP
E3
E2
6K
E1
5'NTR
5'ORF
3'ORF
5'NTR
Non-structural proteins
Structural proteins
E1/E2 (primer)/6K
Genomic + RNA
Capsid

(B)

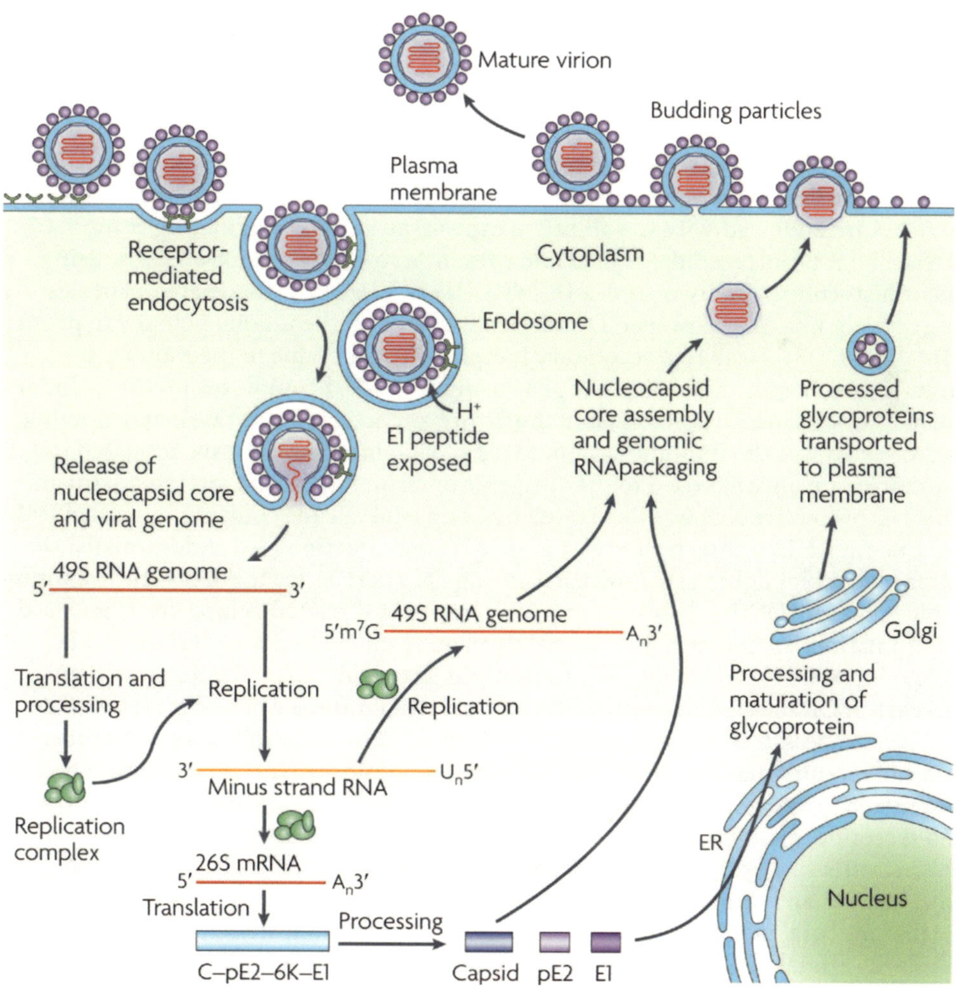
Mature virion
Budding particles
Plasma membrane
Receptor-mediated endocytosis
Cytoplasm
Endosome
H+
E1 peptide exposed
Nucleocapsid core assembly and genomic RNApackaging
Processed glycoproteins transported to plasma membrane
Release of nucleocapsid core and viral genome
49S RNA genome
5'
3'
5'm7G
49S RNA genome
An3'
Golgi
Translation and processing
Replication
Replication
Processing and maturation of glycoprotein
3'
Minus strand RNA
Un5'
Replication complex
ER
26S mRNA
5'
An3'
Nucleus
Translation
Processing
C–pE2–6K–E1
Capsid
pE2
E1

Figure 3.
Chikungunya virus genome structure and infectious cycle. (A) Chikungunya genome structure, (B) chikungunya (CHIK) internalizes within the target cell through receptor mediated endocytosis. Upon entry, CHIK undergo conformational changes leading to E1 peptide exposure as a result of endosomal microenvironment acidity, which favors virus–host cell membrane fusion and subsequent cytoplasmic release of nucleocapsid core and viral genome. Thereafter, two viral mRNA strands are translated to give to two non-structural proteins (nsPs), which are cleaved to generate nsP1–nsP4. The function of the latter are as followed: 1) nsP1 synthesis the negative viral strand RNA and cap it, 2) nsP2 exhibits RNA triphosphatase, helicase and proteinase functions contributing to host cell transcriptional machinery inhibition, 3) nsP3 forms part of the replicase unit and 4) nsP4 exert viral RNA polymerase function. The coordinated activity of these proteins is to produce the viral replication complex, enabling the synthesis of the full-length negative-strand RNA intermediate serving as the precursor to generate the subgenomic (26S) and genomic (49S) RNAs. Once synthesized, the 26S mRNA is translated into C–pE2–6 K–E1 polyprotein precursors, which are further processed by a serine protease to produce a capsid (C), pE2 and E1 glycoproteins. Then, pE2 and E1 assemble in the Golgi and translocate to the plasma membrane, where pE2 is cleaved into E2 (enabling receptor binding) and E3 (ensuring correct pE2 folding and its subsequent assembly with E1). Completion of this viral replication cycle is achieved through 1) assembly of the viral nucleocapsid with the viral RNA, 2) recruitment of membrane-associated envelope glycoproteins and 3) budding at the virus at the host cell membrane [24].

5. CHIKV induced immune response

5.1 The role of innate immunity in chikungunya infection management

The innate immune system refers to the first non-physical and non-specific defense mechanisms to encounter invading pathogens or foreign elements immediately or hours following the appearance of their antigens within the body [29]. To perform its protective role, the host innate immunity relies on antigen-presenting cells (APC) such as macrophages (Mc) and dendritic cells (DC) to neutralize foreign antigens and subsequently present it in a specific way to specialized lymphocytes B (antibody producing cells) and T-cells of the adaptive immunity in secondary lymphoid organs (spleen and ganglions) [30, 31]. Conventionally, all APCs are endowed with the ability to capture an antigen originating from extracellular or intracellular milieu and present it to CD4+ or CD8+ T cells, using major histocompatibility complex II (MHC-II) or I (MHC I) associated peptides respectively [30–32]. However, DCs are endowed with the unique potency to prime CD4+ and CD8+ T-cells (in secondary lymphoid organs) due to their ability to cross-present captured foreign antigens using MHC-II/I complexes [32–34]. Under normal conditions, DC cells exist in immature and inactivated states, hence acting as the sentinel of the immune system [31, 34, 35]. However, DCs are activated into a mature state once exposed to the antigenic determinant of the foreign organism. This DC protective role was illustrated by Long et al., 2013 reporting increased DCs presence at CHIKV infection site 24 and 36 h post infection [36]. Additionally, the latter report highlighted that mice harboring DCs deficiency for dendritic immunogenic receptor (DCIR) displayed more severe CHIKV related symptoms (increased inflammation, edema, weight loss and damage of inoculated foot and the ankle joint) than wild type control [36]. In this line, Das et al., 2015, demonstrated an increase in CD206+ DCs mobilization at the CHIKV infected astrocytes site [37].

Nevertheless, it is well documented that innate immunity following viral infection can recruit inflammatory cells to infected musculoskeletal tissues, with the potential to cause muscular and articular damages inducing the observed pain and discomfort in muscles, joints, and tendons [16]. This CHIKV dependent polyarthritis-like symptoms were reported by Amdekar et al., 2017, to be linked with host inflammatory response regulated by infiltrating macrophages (in joints), T cells, and viral persistence within the immune inaccessible infected sites [38]. Similarly, numerous studies have demonstrated the dichotomic CHIKV reservoir (during chronic infection phase) and modulatory macrophage functions (keeping local Th1/Th2 balance) in the affected tissues (muscles, joints, lymphoid tissues and liver) that they co-infiltrated with mononuclear inflammatory cells [39–41]. These aforementioned results corroborated Gardner et al., 2010 study, revealing the equally important role of macrophages in establishing arthritis symptoms and CHIKV clearance [42]. Furthermore, Phuklia et al., 2013 and Schett, 2007 showed that CHIKV-infected synoviocytes (Cells producing the synovial fluid component important for absorption from the joint cavity and for synovial/blood fluid exchange) were able to promote the migration and differentiation of both monocytes and macrophages into joints damaging osteoclast-like cells, capable of producing high levels of arthritis mediators (Interleukin-6 and Tumor Necrosis Factor-α) [43, 44]. In contrast, Haist et al., 2017, underlined the protective role of inflammatory Ly6C^{hi} CCR2+ monocytes in controlling CHIKV infectious, as their depletion (using diphtheria toxin on CCR2-DTR^{+} mice) was associated with severe disease symptoms and reduction in Ly6C and NK cells in bloodstream and muscles when compared to wild type mice [45].

6. Chikungunya and adaptive immunity

Humoral and cell-mediated immunity hold the center stage for protection against CHIKV infection through the combined action of T and B-lymphocytes, respectively [46]. Multiple human and animal studies have demonstrated the host immune system's ability to induce the production of neutralizing anti-CHIKV antibodies, to rapidly clear CHIKV viral loads and establish long-term immunity [1, 10, 46]. This adaptive humoral immunity relies on immunoglobulin-M (IgM: representing ~30% of circulating antibodies) to primarily entrap the CHIKV antigen to secondary lymphoid tissues by bridging the innate and adaptive immunity before the onset of the robust and specific life-long protecting IgG response [1, 47]. During the chikungunya fever acute phase, neutralizing IgM are produced as early as 2–6 days post-infection and act to reduce viral loads (**Figure 4**) [48]. This neutralizing IgM capacity perdures up to 10 days following CHIKV infection before synergizing with specific IgG response [1]. Interestingly, Couderc and Lecuit et al.,2015 reported persistent anti-CHIKV IgM in chronic chikungunya fever patients related to repeated CHIKV antigen and RNA exposure [49]. Of late, Tanabe et al., 2018 showed that IgM antibodies preferentially interact with cognate E1-E2 fusion glycoprotein epitopes found on CHIKV outer surface [23, 46] and that long term viral immune protection was achieved through specific IgG production, persisting up to 19 years following the first infectious episode (1991 Thailand CHIKV outbreak) [50]. Among all IgG subtypes, IgG3 was found to be the most predominant, able to serve as a predictive marker of high-risk patients (when minimally produced) or as a prophylactic agent, able to passively transfer from mother to newborn via the placenta and limit viral metastases to distant muscles and joints [1]. This pentameric immunoglobulin structure armed them with the ability to easily mediate CHIKV aggregation, recognition and elimination by cytotoxic CD8+ T cells [46]. Unfortunately, CD4+ T-cells can be detrimental to CHIKV infected mice, as it was reported by Theo et al., 2017 that they can severely damage the joints of T-cell receptor-deficient mice when adoptively transferred [46, 51]. Mitigation of these undesired CD4+ T-cell effects could be performed using fingolimod (phosphorylated sphingosine 1-phosphate receptor 1 agonist: S1PR1) treatment, blocking S1PR1 mediated CD4+ T-cells dissemination to the joints of CHIKV infected mice [46, 51]. In a parallel study, Miner et al., 2017 demonstrated the synergy of immunosuppressive cytotoxic T-lymphocyte-antigen-4 (CTLA-4) abatacept (blocking CD4 co-stimulatory activating signals) with anti-CHIKV (reducing viral load) in controlling arthritis and CHIKV infection, respectively [52]. This result was

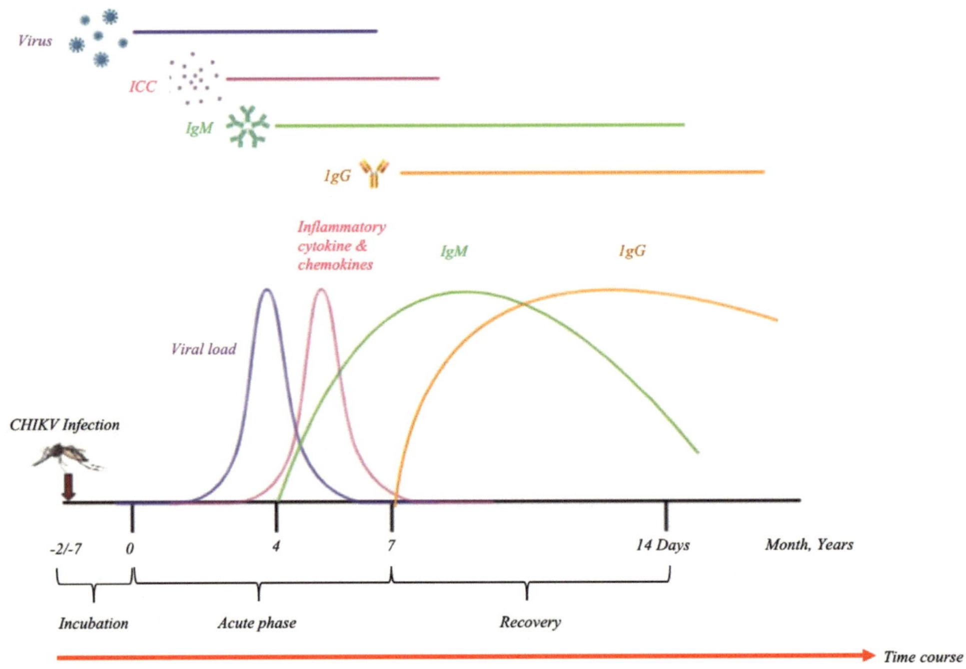

Figure 4.
CHIKV infection and immune response: CHIKV infection begin with mosquito's bites, allowing viral entry into serum and subsequent dissemination into peripheral organs (lymphoid, muscles and joints), leading to the onset of symptoms (acute phase) that can perdure beyond 8 days. During the acute phase (0–4 days), neutralizing IgMs are produced, and their increase inversely correlates with CHIKV viral loads. During the recovery phase or convalescence (beyond 7 days), IgGs are produced and act in concert with IgM to provide long-term immune protection.

particularly relevant, as it may pave the way for novel antibody therapeutic strategies, with the potential to clinically benefit CHIKV infected patients.

7. Chikungunya virus therapeutic treatment and future perspectives

Targeted antibody-based immunotherapy was developed to address the unmet CHIKV therapeutic clinical needs [1]. In this regard, immunotherapy using IgG has widely been developed and has demonstrated the potential to reach clinical fruition by exerting its virucidal (Virus killing activity) and prophylactic activities on infected patients [1]. This IgG virucidal effect was confirmed by Scott et al., 2017 showing its ability to induce complete recovery in encephalitis infected patients, using a therapeutic dose of 400 mg/kg for 5 days [2]. With this in mind, Fernandes et al., 2019 corroborated these latter results, by achieving a 10 day total recovery, following a combination therapy involving antibiotic and IgG treatment (400 mg/kg for 5 days) on a severely infected 56 years old patient, presenting with atypical dermatological form associated with edema and hemorrhagic bullous skin lesions [53]. This IgG immunotherapeutic agent could either be used to immunized healthy or asymptomatic individuals in endemic areas (with the aim to reduce CHIKV propagation) or to treat high-risk patients such as pregnant women, newborns, immunocompromised individuals, elders or patients with preexisting arthritis [1]. For example, Couderc et al. 2009 demonstrated the therapeutic and prophylactic actions of IgGs (purified from convalescent CHIKV infected donor), protecting adult immunocompromised and immunocompetent mice neonates from CHIKV re-challenge and severe neurological symptoms associated with chronic CHIKV infection [54]. Based on these accumulative reports, a phase I/II clinical trial was initiated to evaluate the therapeutic and prophylactic efficacy of CHIKV IgG therapy to newborns of mothers with acute CHIKV infection, whose infectious rates reached 49% (Clinical trials: NCT02230163) [14]. However, the efficacy of CHIKV IgG immunotherapy can be compromised by immune evasion, arising from monoclonal Abs (mAbs) selective pressure or accumulated genetic mutations able to suppress antigen specificity, thus antigen–antibody interaction [1]. With the advent of recombinant antibody engineering technology, efforts to overcome these unwanted effects were developed and led to the generation of bispecific antibodies that can recognize two or more epitopes; a detailed discussion beyond the scope of this review has been provided by Nyakatura et al., 2017 [55]. Besides immune evasion, other factors like antibody-dependent enhancement (ADE), characterized by sub-neutralizing Abs concentration that is permissive for viral replication, has been identified as a major challenge for CHIKV management [1, 56]. In spite of the single serotype status of CHIKV, ADE cannot be overlooked with respect to CHIKV reemergence, as it has been observed in other viral diseases, including Dengue, Rabies virus, influenza and HIV [1]. Also, antibody-based therapy is generally associated with high production costs, which may restrain therapeutic usage due to affordability. To address these issues, nucleic acid vaccines made up of mRNA or

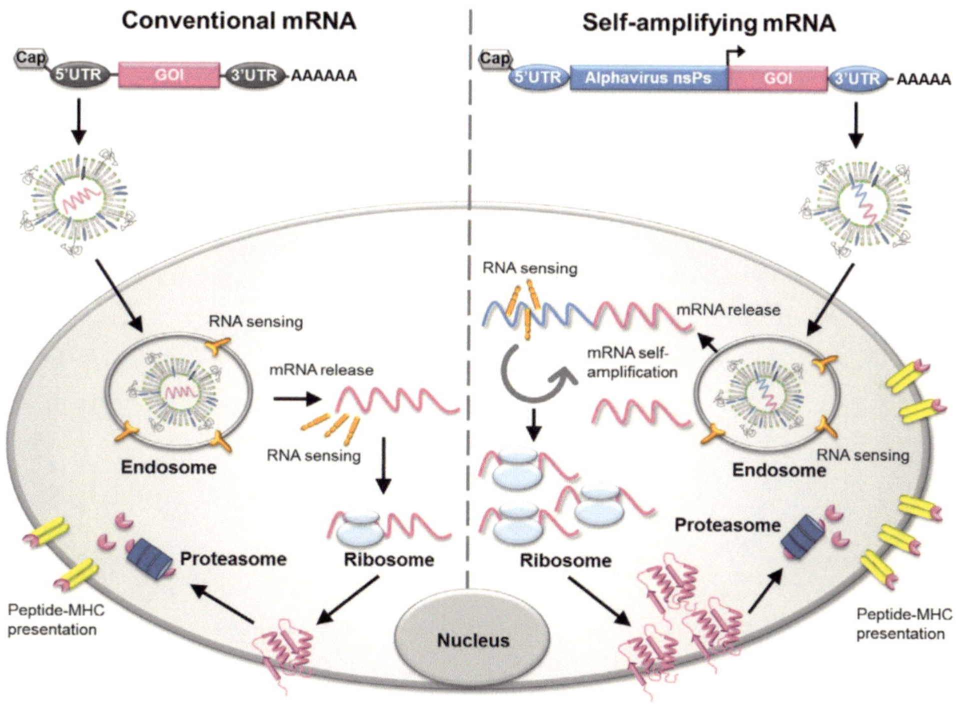

Figure 5.
mRNA vaccine mechanism of action. Conventional mRNA possesses disease specific gene of interest (GOI) encoding the antigen DNA sequence that is respectively capped at the 5′ end and polyadenylated (poly-a tail) at the 3′ untranslated region (UTR). Upon internalization within the host cell, viral mRNA is released from the endosome to the cytosol, where it is immediately translated by the ribosomes and post-translationally modified by the proteasome. In opposition to the conventional mRNA vaccination, the self-amplifying mRNA method mostly uses positive-sense single-stranded viral RNA encoding the disease specific antigen and viral nonstructural proteins (nsPs) driving intracellular RNA amplification and significant antigen expression. These two vaccination methods need a delivery system for host cell internalization, commonly performed through endocytosis, preceding cytosolic viral mRNA cargo releases from the endosome, driving translation and subsequent viral antigen protein processing for MHC presentation to ensue and activate host immunity [59].

plasmid DNA (pDNA) were developed [57, 58]. These novel vaccines are commonly used to treat mRNA alphavirus and are mainly produced by genetically substituting viral encoding structural protein with target antigen encoding genes while preserving the RNA replication machinery [57]. Hence, when injected into patients, these vaccines (mRNA) mimic the virus by taking advantage of the host cell machinery to efficiently transcribe an antigen encoded RNA into an antigen encoded DNA, which is subsequently translated and post-translationally modified into a form (protein) that resemble the natural antigen that can successively stimulate and activate the innate and adaptive immunity (**Figure 5**) [57, 58]. Recently, Kose et al. (2019) demonstrated CHIKV and arthritis protecting properties of an infused nanoparticle encoding CHIKV antibody mRNA, which was as good as purified IgG mAbs in stimulating protective anti-CHIKV serum concentrations in macaques [60].

So far, there are no clinically approved RNA vaccines to treat human diseases. Yet, in response to the ongoing coronavirus disease 2019 (COVID-19) pandemic, multiple clinical trials such as NCT04283461, have been initiated to test the safety of an mRNA vaccine (encoding SARS-CoV-2 spike protein), which successfully produced SARS-CoV-2 antibodies and had no clinically adverse effects [61, 62]. Currently, it has progressed into phase III clinical trial (NCT04470427) to evaluate its efficacy against COVID-19. Likewise, other clinical trials are presently investigating the safety, tolerability and immunogenicity of zika virus envelop protein encoded mRNA vaccines (NCT04064905; NCT03014089) [61, 63]. Taken altogether, it becomes evident that the rapid advances made in recombinant DNA technology, will revolutionize the way we approach and promptly respond to endemic CHIKV/COVID-19 like diseases.

Author details

Fleury Augustin Nsole Biteghe[1*†], Chalomie Nyangone Ekome Toung[2], Jean De La Croix Ndong[3], Neelakshi Mungra[4], Tahir B. Dar[1] and Arnaud John Kombe Kombe[5†]

1 Department of Radiation Oncology and Biomedical Sciences, Cedars-Sinai Medical, Los Angeles, USA

2 Zhongshan Medical School, Sun Yat-Sen University, Guangzhou, China

3 Federated Departments of Biological Sciences, Rutgers University School of Arts and Science, USA

4 Faculty of Health Sciences, Medical Biotechnology and Immunotherapy Research Unit, Institute of Infectious Disease and Molecular Medicine, University of Cape Town, Cape Town, South Africa

5 Division of Molecular Medicine, Hefei National Laboratory for Physical Sciences at Microscale, CAS Key Laboratory of Innate Immunity and Chronic Disease, Division of Life Sciences and Medicine, University of Science and Technology of China, Hefei, China

*Address all correspondence to: fleury.nsolebiteghe@cshs.org

†Both authors equally contributed

References

[1] Kumar R, Shrivastava T, Samal S, Ahmed S, Parray HA. Antibody-based therapeutic interventions: possible strategy to counter chikungunya viral infection. Appl Microbiol Biotechnol. 2020;104(8):3209-28.

[2] Scott SS de O, Braga-Neto P, Pereira LP, Nóbrega PR, de Assis Aquino Gondim F, Sobreira-Neto MA, et al. Immunoglobulin-responsive chikungunya encephalitis: two case reports. J Neurovirol. 2017;23(4):625-31.

[3] MC R. An epidemic of virus disease in Southern Province, Tanganyika Territory, in 1952-53. Trans R Soc Trop Med Hyg. 1955;49(1):28-32.

[4] Thiboutot MM, Kannan S, Kawalekar OU, Shedlock DJ, Khan AS, Sarangan G et al. Chikungunya: a potentially emerging epidemic? PLoS Negl Trop Dis. 2010;4(4):e63.

[5] SB H. Reappearance of chikungunya, formerly called dengue, in the Americas. Emerg Infect Dis. 2015;21(4):557-61.

[6] Halstead SB. Reappearance of chikungunya, formerly called Dengue, in the Americas. Emerg Infect Dis. 2015;21(4):557-61.

[7] Clayton AM. Monoclonal antibodies as prophylactic and therapeutic agents against chikungunya virus. J Infect Dis. 2016;214(Suppl 5):S506-9.

[8] Gopalan, S.S.; Das A. Household economic impact of an emerging disease in terms of catastrophic out-of-pocket health care expenditure and loss of productivity: Investigation of an outbreak of chikungunya in orissa, india. J Vector Borne Dis. 2009;46:57-64.

[9] Jin J, Simmons G. Antiviral functions of monoclonal antibodies against chikungunya virus. Viruses. 2019;11(4):1-17.

[10] Powers AM. Vaccine and therapeutic options to control chikungunya virus. Clin Microbiol Rev. 2018;31(1):1-29.

[11] Burt FJ, Chen W, Miner JJ, Lenschow DJ, Merits A, Schnettler E, Kohl A, Rudd PA, TaylorA, Herrero LJ, ZaidA, NgLFP MS. Chikungunya virus: an update on the biology and pathogenesis of this emerging pathogen. Lancet Infect Dis. 2017;17(4):e107-17.

[12] Marston HD, Paules CI FA. Monoclonal antibodies for emerging infectious diseases - borrowing from history. N Engl J Med 3781469-1472. 2018;378:1469-72.

[13] Gerardin P, Samperiz S, Ramful D, Boumahni B, Bintner M, Alessandri JL et al. Neurocognitive outcome of children exposed to perinatal mother-to-child Chikungunya virus infection: the CHIMERE cohort study on Reunion Island. PLoS Negl Trop Dis. 2014;8(7): e2996.

[14] Cardona-Correa SE, Castaño-Jaramillo LM, Quevedo-Vélez A. Vertical transmission of chikungunya virus infection. Case report. Rev Chil Pediatr. 2017;88(2):285-8.

[15] Burt FJ, Rolph MS, Rulli NE, Mahalingam S, Heise MT. Chikungunya: A re-emerging virus. In: The Lancet. Elsevier; 2012. p. 662-71.

[16] Silva LA, Dermody TS. Chikungunya virus: Epidemiology, replication, disease mechanisms, and prospective intervention strategies. J Clin Invest. 2017;127(3):737-49.

[17] Silva LA DT. Chikungunya virus: epidemiology, replication, disease mechanisms, and prospective intervention strategies. J Clin Invest. 2017;127(3):737-49.

[18] 1. Moizéis RNC, Fernandes TAA de M, Guedes PM da M, Pereira HWB, Lanza DCF, Azevedo JWV de et al. Chikungunya fever: a threat to global public health. Pathog Glob Heal. 2018;112(4):182-94.

[19] Sa PKO, Nunes MM, Leite IR, Campelo M, Leao CFR, Souza JR, Castellano LR FA(. Chikungunya virus infection with severe neurologic manifestations: report offour fatal cases. Rev Soc Bras Med Trop. 2017;50: 265-2687.

[20] Josseran L, Paquet C, Zehgnoun A, Caillere N, Le Tertre A, Solet JL LM. Chikungunya disease outbreak, Reunion Island. Emerg Infect Dis. 2006;12: 1994-5.

[21] Weaver SC, Osorio JE, Livengood JA, Chen R SD. Chikungunya virus and prospects for a vaccine. Expert Rev Vaccines. 2012;11(9):1087-101.

[22] Weaver SC, Osorio JE, Livengood JA, Chen R, Dan T, Weaver SC, et al. Chikungunya virus and prospects for a vaccine Chikungunya virus and prospects for a vaccine. Expert Rev Vaccines. 2012;11(9):1087-101.

[23] Reddy V, Desai A, Krishna SS, Vasanthapuram R. Molecular Mimicry between Chikungunya Virus and Host Components: A Possible Mechanism for the Arthritic Manifestations. PLoS Negl Trop Dis. 2017;11(1):1-20.

[24] Schwartz O, Albert ML. Biology and pathogenesis of chikungunya virus. Nat Rev Microbiol. 2010;8(7):491-500.

[25] Moizéis RNC, Fernandes TAA de M, Guedes PM da M, Pereira HWB, Lanza DCF, Azevedo JWV de, et al. Chikungunya fever: a threat to global public health. Pathog Glob Health. 2018;112(4):182-94.

[26] Das T et al. Chikungunya fever: CNS infection and pathologies of a re-emerging arbovirus. Prog Neurobiol. 2010;91(2):121-9.

[27] Rosso F, Rodriguez S, Cedano JA, Mora BL, Moncada PA VJ(. Chikungunya in solid organ transplant recipients, a case se- ries and literature review. Transpl Infect Dis. 2018;20(6):e12978.

[28] Campos GS, Albuquerque Bandeira AC, Diniz Rocha VF, Dias JP, Carvalho RH SS. First detection of chikungunya virus in breast milk. Pediatr Infect Dis J. 2017;36(10):1015-7.

[29] Dar TB, Henson RM, Shiao SL. Targeting innate immunity to enhance the efficacy of radiation therapy. Front Immunol. 2019;9:1-11.

[30] Woo S-R, Corrales L, Gajewski TF. Innate Immune Recognition of Cancer. Annu Rev Immunol. 2015;33(1):445-74.

[31] Patente TA, Pinho MP, Oliveira AA, Evangelista GCM, Bergami-Santos PC, Barbuto JAM. Human dendritic cells: Their heterogeneity and clinical application potential in cancer immunotherapy. Front Immunol. 2019;9(3176):1-18.

[32] Garg AD, Coulie PG, Van den Eynde BJ, Agostinis P. Integrating Next-Generation Dendritic Cell Vaccines into the Current Cancer Immunotherapy Landscape. Vol. 38, Trends in Immunology. Elsevier Ltd; 2017. p. 577-93.

[33] Cance JC, Crozat K, Dalod M, Mattiuz R. Are conventional type 1 dendritic cells critical for protective antitomor immunity and how? Front Immunol. 2019;10(FEB).

[34] Bol KF, Schreibelt G, Gerritsen WR, De Vries IJM, Figdor CG. Dendritic cell-based immunotherapy: State of the art and beyond. Clin Cancer Res. 2016;22(8):1897-906.

[35] Shang N, Figini M, Shangguan J, Wang B, Sun C, Pan L, et al. Dendritic cells based immunotherapy. Vol. 27, Cel l Research. E-Century Publishing Corporation; 2017. p. 74-95.

[36] Long KM, Whitmore AC, Ferris MT, Sempowski GD, McGee C, Trollinger B, et al. Dendritic Cell Immunoreceptor Regulates Chikungunya Virus Pathogenesis in Mice. J Virol. 2013;87(10):5697-706.

[37] Das T, Hoarau JJ, Bandjee MCJ, Marianne M, Gasque P. Multifaceted innate immune responses engaged by astrocytes, microglia and resident dendritic cells against Chikungunya neuroinfection. J Gen Virol. 2015;96(2):294-310.

[38] Sarika Amdekar, Deepti Parashar and KA. Chikungunya Virus-Induced Arthritis: Role of Host and Viral Factors in the Pathogenesis. Viral immunoogy. 2017;30(10):691-702.

[39] Labadie, K., Larcher, T., Joubert, C., Mannioui, A., Delache, B., Brochard, P. et al. Chikungunya disease in nonhuman primates involves long-term viral persistence in macrophages. (J Clin Invest. 2010;120:894-906.

[40] Dupuis-Maguiraga, L., Noret, M., Brun, S., Le Grand, R., Gras, G., and Roques P. Chikungunya disease: infection-associated markers from the acute to the chronic phase of arbovirus-induced arthralgia. PLoS Negl Trop Dis. 2012;6:e1446.

[41] Ziegler, S. A., Lu, L., da Rosa, A. P., Xiao, S. Y., and Tesh RB. An animal model for studying the pathogenesis of chikungunya virus infection. Am J Trop Med. 2008;79:133-9.

[42] Gardner J, Anraku I, Le TT, Larcher T, Major L, Roques P, et al. Chikungunya Virus Arthritis in Adult Wild-Type Mice. J Virol. 2010;84(16):8021-32.

[43] Phuklia, W., Kasisith, J., Modhiran, N., Rodpai, E., Thannagith, M., Thongsakulprasert, T. et al. Osteoclastogenesis induced by CHIKV-infected fibroblast-like synoviocytes: a possible interplay between synoviocytes and monocytes/macrophages in CHIKV-induced arthralgia/arthritis. Virus Res. 2013;177:179-88.

[44] Schett G. Cells of the synovium in rheumatoid arthritis. Osteoclasts. Arthritis Res Ther. 2007;9(1):1-6.

[45] Haist KC, Burrack KS, Davenport BJ, Morrison TE. Inflammatory monocytes mediate control of acute alphavirus infection in mice. PLoS Pathog. 2017;13(12):1-30.

[46] Tanabe ISB, Tanabe ELL, Santos EC, Martins W V., Araújo IMTC, Cavalcante MCA, et al. Cellular and Molecular Immune Response to Chikungunya Virus Infection. Front Cell Infect Microbiol. 2018;8(October):345.

[47] Vollmers HP BS. The "early birds": natural IgM antibod- ies and immune surveillance. Histol Histopathol. 2005;20(3):927-37.

[48] Petitdemange C, Wauquier N V V. Control ofimmunopa- thology during chikungunya virus infection. J Allergy Clin Immunol. 2015;135(4):846-55.

[49] Couderc T LM. Chikungunya virus pathogenesis: from bed- side to bench. Antivir Res. 2015;121:120-31.

[50] Nitatpattana N, Kanjanopas K, Yoksan S, Satimai W, Vongba N, Langdatsuwan S, Nakgoi K, Ratchakum S, Wauquier N, Souris M, Auewarakul P GJ. Long-term persistence of chikungunya virus neutralizing antibodies in human populations of north eastern Thailand. Virol J. 2014;11:183.

[51] Teo, T. H., Chan, Y. H., Lee, W. W., Lum, F. M., Amrun, S. N., Her, Z. et al.

Fingolimod treatment abrogates chikungunya virus-induced arthralgia. Sci Transl Med. 2017;9(375):eaal1333.

[52] Miner JJ, Cook LE, Hong JP, Smith AM, Richner JM, Shimak RM, Young AR, Monte K, Poddar S, Crowe JE Jr, Lenschow DJ DM. Therapy with CTLA4-Ig and an antiviral monoclonal antibody controls chikungunya virus arthritis. Sci Transl Med. 2017;9(375):eaah3438.

[53] Fernandes AI V., Souza JR, Silva AR, Cruz SBSC, Castellano LRC. Immunoglobulin therapy in a patient with severe chikungunya fever and vesiculobullous lesions. Front Immunol. 2019;10(JUL):1-6.

[54] Couderc T, Khandoudi N, GrandadamM, Visse C, Gangneux N, Bagot S, Prost JF LM. Prophylaxis and therapy for chikungunya virus infection. J Infect Dis. 2009;Couderc T, (4):516-23.

[55] Nyakatura EK, Soare AY, Lai JR. Bispecific antibodies for viral immunotherapy. Hum Vaccines Immunother. 2017;13(4):836-42.

[56] Lum FM, Couderc T, Chia BS, Ong RY, Her Z, Chow A, Leo YS, Kam YW, Renia L, Lecuit M NL. Antibody-mediated en- hancement aggravates chikungunya virus infection and disease severity. Sci Rep. 2018;8(1):1860.

[57] Pitman MC, Lau JSY MJ et al. Barriers and strategies to achieve a cure for HIV. lancet HIV. 2018;5(317-28).

[58] Dharanidharan Ramamurthy, Trishana Nundalall, Sanele Cingo, Neelakshi Mungra, Maryam Karaan, Krupa Naran1 SB. Recent Advances in Immunotherapies Against Infectious Diseases. Immunother Adv. 2020;1-6.

[59] Maruggi G, Zhang C, Li J, Ulmer JB, Yu D. mRNA as a Transformative Technology for Vaccine Development to Control Infectious Diseases. Mol Ther. 2019;27(4):757-72. Available from: https://doi.org/10.1016/j.ymthe.2019.01.020

[60] Kose N, Fox JM, Sapparapu G, Bombardi R, Tennekoon RN, de Silva AD, Elbashir SM, Theisen MA, Humphris-Narayanan E, Ciaramella G, Himansu S, Diamond MS CJJ. A lipid-encapsulated mRNA encoding a potently neutralizing human monoclonal antibody protects against chikungunya infection. Sci Immunol. 2019;4(35):eaaw6647.

[61] Kim YC, Dema B, Reyes-Sandoval A. COVID-19 vaccines: breaking record times to first-in-human trials. npj Vaccines. 2020;5(1):19-21.

[62] Tung Thanh Le, Zacharias Andreadakis, Arun Kumar, Raúl Gómez Román, Stig Tollefsen, Melanie Saville SM. The COVID-19 vaccine development landscape. Nat Rev Drug Discov. 2020;19(5):305-6.

[63] Jackson NAC, Kester KE, Casimiro D, Gurunathan S, DeRosa F. The promise of mRNA vaccines: a biotech and industrial perspective. npj Vaccines. 2020;5(1):3-8.